Electrocardiogram Interpretation and Emergency Intervention

CARLOS S. SARAD
1363 ROSS ROAD
NORTH VANCOUVER BC
CANADA V7J 1V3

Electrocardiogram Interpretation and Emergency Intervention

Madeline Dignan Fassler, RN, BSN, CEN
Clinical Education Coordinator
Kaiser Permanente Medical Center
Hayward, California
President
Creative Education Resources, Inc.
San Leadro, California

Barbara Tueller Steuble, RN, MS, CEN
Assistant Professor of Nursing
Samuel Merritt College
Oakland, California
Staff Nurse, ICU and Shift Supervisor
Amador Hospital
Jackson, California

Springhouse Corporation
Springhouse, Pennsylvania

Staff

Executive Director, Editorial
Stanley Loeb

Director of Trade and Textbooks
Minnie B. Rose, RN, BSN, MEd

Art Director
John Hubbard

Senior Acquisitions Editor
Susan L. Mease

Drug Information Editor
George J. Blake, RPh, MS

Editor
David Moreau

Copy Editors
Mary Durkin, Mary Hohenhaus Hardy

Design
Diehl Design

Illustration
Greg Purdone (cover), Bob Jackson

Manufacturing
Deborah Meiris (manager), T.A. Landis, Jennifer Suter

Library of Congress Cataloging-in-Publication Data

Fassler, Madeline Dignan.
  Electrocardiograminterpretation and emergency intervention / Madeline Dignan Fassler, Barbara Tueller Steuble.
    p. cm.
  Includes bibliographical references and index.
  ISBN 0-87434-334-8
  1. Electrocardiography. 2. Heart--Diseases. 3. Medical emergencies. 4. Heart--Diseases--Nursing. I. Steuble, Barbara Tueller. II. Title.
  [DNLM: 1. Arrhythmia--diagnosis. 2. Arrhythmia--therapy. 3. Emergencies. 4. Electrocardiography. WG 205 F249e]
RC683.5.E5F28 1991
616.1'207547--dc20
DNLM/DLC   91-4602
                                                    CIP

Printed in the United States of America.

ECG1-021192

Contents

Acknowledgments

We wish to express our gratitude to the nurses and students who have attended our courses and shared their experiences and ideas with us; to our educator colleagues and co-instructors of ACLS courses for their ideas and critiques; to Samuel Merritt College, Oakland, California; and to Kaiser Permanente Medical Center, Hayward, California, especially the ICU and ER staff nurses.

Dedication

To Mike, Tim, Brian, Missy, and Conan for their patience and understanding

M.D.F.

To my husband, Roger H. Steuble, for his support, encouragement, and love

B.T.S.

Preface

An elderly woman with asystole, a middle-aged businessman with complete heart block, a 3-week-old infant with supraventricular tachycardia—in the past, such patients were treated only in hospitals, primarily by cardiac experts who had had years of intensive training in their specialty. More recently, however, greater numbers of health care professionals—including nurses and paramedics—have become directly involved in managing cardiac emergencies, both within and outside the traditional hospital setting. Indeed, advanced cardiac life support (ACLS) certification from the American Heart Association is becoming a mandatory requirement for nursing practice not only in emergency departments, coronary care units, and operating rooms but also in outpatient clinics and day hospitals.

Such widespread involvement of nurses and other health care professionals demands that they possess keen assessment skills, extensive knowledge of standard treatment principles, and the wherewithal to intervene quickly in a life-threatening crisis. Unfortunately, much of the literature written for nonphysicians focuses too heavily on rhythm interpretation, slighting essential therapeutic and emergency interventions based on the interpretation. *Electrocardiogram Interpretation and Emergency Intervention* bridges that gap, balancing a detailed discussion of rhythm interpretation with extensive coverage of currently accepted ACLS treatment standards.

Chapter 1 provides a brief review of cardiac anatomy and physiology, looking at the heart's location and structures; the cardiac cycle; pulmonary, systemic, and coronary circulation; hemodynamics; cardiac innervation; and the heart's conduction system.

Chapter 2 explains electrophysiology and electrocardiogram (ECG) basics—depolarization and repolarization, transmembrane action potentials, properties of cardiac cells, ECG characteristics, normal complexes, and lead placement.

Chapter 3 explores the 12-lead ECG, reviewing axis determination, ventricular activation, ischemia, injury, myocardial infarction patterns, interventricular conduction delays, bundle branch blocks and aberrations, preexcitation syndromes, and drug and electrolyte effects on cellular electrophysiology.

Chapter 4 presents pertinent ECG strips to accompany discussions of asystole and atrioventricular (AV) blocks as well as rhythms originating in the sinus node (sinus rhythm, sinus bradycardia, sinus tachycardia, sinus arrest, and sinoatrial block), atria (premature atrial complex, atrial tachycardia, atrial flutter, and atrial fibrillation), AV junction (premature junctional complex, junctional rhythm, and supraventricular tachycardia), and ventricles (premature ventricular complex, idioventricular rhythm, accelerated ventricular rhythm, ventricular tachycardia, torsades de pointes, and ventricular fibrillation).

Chapter 5 details the benefits of inotropic and vasoactive drugs, sympathetic and parasympathetic blocking agents, antiarrhythmics, and miscellaneous drugs, complete with indications, dosages, and precautions.

Chapter 6 highlights electrical and mechanical interventions—cardiopulmonary resuscitation, defibrillation, cardioversion, precordial thump, and pacemaker therapy.

Chapters 7 to 13 cover the standard emergency interventions for ventricular fibrillation, ventricular tachycardia, ventricular asystole, electromechanical dissociation, paroxysmal supraventricular tachycardia, atrial fibrillation, bradycardias, AV blocks, and ventricular ectopy.

Chapter 14 examines cardiac emergencies that can develop in pediatric patients and the special interventions they require.

The book includes many special features to facilitate learning. Nearly 200 ECG strips on virtually every type of normal and abnormal heart rhythm accompany text discussions of both interpretation and intervention. Anatomical drawings, diagrams, charts, and graphs appear throughout the text to illustrate key concepts and enhance the reader's understanding of complex material. The chapters devoted to emergency interventions for arrhythmias contain easy-to-follow algorithms (also called decision trees) that guide the reader, step by step, through actions to take during the crisis. Several scenarios (case studies) follow each algorithm, thus reinforcing the specific interventions in various contexts. These scenarios (shown in *italic* type) integrate patient signs and symptoms, assessment findings, and supporting laboratory data with appropriate interventions from the health care team (signalled by the algorithm logo in the left margin). Rationales follow each intervention in a scenario, clearly explaining the purpose of every intervention. Study questions and answers at the end of these chapters—as well as a Self-Test appendix—promote content recall and enable the reader to identify knowledge strengths and pinpoint areas that may require additional study. Finally, selected references provide ample suggestions for further investigation of relevant topics.

Electrocardiogram Interpretation and Emergency Intervention is an invaluable reference for nurses, physicians, paramedics, and other health care professionals who provide emergency cardiac care. The book offers particular advantages to ACLS course participants who want to review the content for theoretical and practical testing areas. Instructors can also use the book as a springboard for providing realistic teaching and testing situations to develop their students' decision-making and problem-solving skills. Ultimately, of course, we hope this book enhances the quality of emergency cardiac care performed by all health care professionals.

Madeline Dignan Fassler
Barbara Tueller Steuble

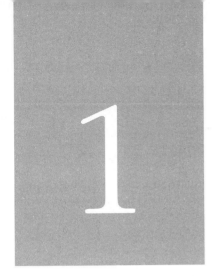

1

The Heart: Anatomy and Physiology

Accurate electrocardiogram interpretation and timely interventions during cardiac emergencies require a sound understanding of heart function and pump dynamics. This chapter provides a brief review of cardiac structures; the cardiac cycle; pulmonary, systemic, and coronary circulation; hemodynamics; cardiac innervation; and the cardiac conduction system.

Cardiac location and structures

The heart is the driving force of the circulatory system, contracting about 70 times/minute to pump an adequate volume of blood with sufficient pressure to perfuse all body organs and tissues. The muscular organ, about the size of a clenched fist, weighs from 300 to 400 g. It is located within the mediastinum of the thoracic cavity, above the diaphragm and between the lungs. This location subjects the heart's activity to influence from all pressure variances during respiration.

LOCATION OF CARDIAC STRUCTURES

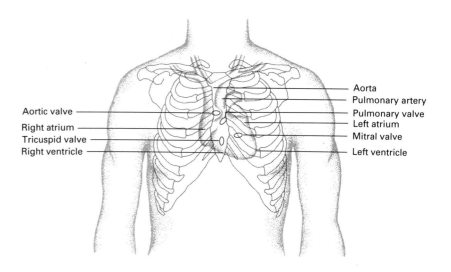

Aortic valve
Right atrium
Tricuspid valve
Right ventricle

Aorta
Pulmonary artery
Pulmonary valve
Left atrium
Mitral valve
Left ventricle

Intrathoracic pressure varies with the respiratory cycle. On inspiration, the heart moves slightly vertically, and the increased negative pressure generated in the thoracic cavity increases venous blood return to the heart and pulmonary blood flow. On expiration, the heart moves slightly horizontally as the diaphragm rises, and a decreased negative pressure is generated.

The pericardial sac is a fibrous membrane that doubles over onto itself to form two surfaces. A small amount of pericardial fluid in the sac allows the two surfaces to slide over each other without friction as the heart beats. The pericardium performs several functions. First, it provides shock-absorbing protection. Second, it acts as a protective barrier against bacterial invasion from the lungs. Third, because of its fibrous nature, it protects the heart from sudden overdistention and increase in size.

The heart has three tissue layers: the epicardium (outer layer), the myocardium (middle layer), and the endocardium (inner layer). The epicardium is the thin inner layer of the pericardium. The myocardium, thickest of the three layers, is composed of muscle fibers that contract, creating the pumping effect of cardiac activity. The endocardium, a smooth, membranous layer that lines all cardiac chambers and valve leaflets, is continuous with the intima, or lining, of the aorta and arteries.

The heart's four chambers—the right and left atria and the right and left ventricles—are separated by the interatrial and interventricular septa. The atria are thin-walled, low-pressure chambers that serve primarily as reservoirs for blood flow into the ventricles. The ventricles are formed by muscle fibers that contract to eject blood to the pulmonary vasculature (right) and systemic circulation (left). Because the left ventricle must achieve the high pressure needed for systemic circulation, it is much thicker than the right ventricle.

BLOOD FLOW THROUGH THE HEART

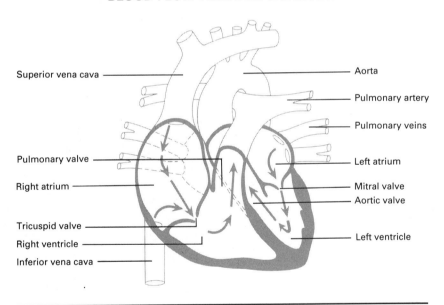

The right atrium receives venous blood from the body via the venae cavae. The superior vena cava returns blood from the structures above the diaphragm, and the inferior vena cava drains venous blood from below the diaphragm. The coronary sinus returns venous blood to the right atrium. At the base of the right atrium is the tricuspid valve, which controls blood flow into the right ventricle and prevents back flow to the atrium during ventricular systole. The right ventricle pumps blood through the pulmonary valve and the branches of the pulmonary artery to the lobes of the lungs, the pulmonary capillaries, and the alveolar capillaries that surround the alveoli.

At the alveolar capillaries, gas exchange occurs; that is, blood gives off carbon dioxide and receives oxygen. Then, oxygenated blood returns through the pulmonary veins to the left atrium. The mitral valve at the base of the left atrium controls blood flow to the left ventricle and prevents backflow to the left atrium. Both the mitral and the tricuspid valves are attached to the strong chordae tendineae, fibrous filaments that arise from the papillary muscles of the ventricle and work to prevent eversion of the valves when the ventricle contracts. The left ventricle pumps blood through the aortic valve into the aorta.

The basic contractile unit in the myocardium, the sarcomere, is composed of actin and myosin filaments, which are contractile proteins. The degree to which actin and myosin overlap depends on the length of the sarcomere, which is determined by muscle stretch. Less overlap occurs during diastole, as the ventricle fills and the muscle stretches; more overlap occurs during systole, when the muscle contracts. Contraction occurs when the action potential stimulates movement of calcium ions to binding sites on the actin filaments. This movement, combined with energy release, causes the filaments to slide past each other and shorten the sarcomere.

Cardiac cycle

The heart ejects blood during ventricular systole, which comprises approximately one-third of the cardiac cycle. The cardiac muscles relax during diastole, which comprises the remaining two-thirds of the cardiac cycle. The first phase of systole, called *isovolumetric contraction,* begins with closure of the tricuspid and mitral valves. Pressure in the walls of the ventricles builds in preparation for mechanical contraction. When ventricular pressure becomes higher than pressure in the aorta and pulmonary artery, the pulmonary and aortic valves open, allowing for rapid ejection of blood. Blood is ejected rapidly at first and then more slowly as pressure decreases. Pressure in the ventricles continues to fall until the aortic and pulmonary valves close. Closure of the valves begins the first phase of diastole, called *isovolumetric relaxation.* During this time, ventricular pressure continues to decrease. When pressure in the ventricles becomes less than atrial pressure, the tricuspid and mitral valves open, permitting rapid ventricular filling. The ventricle continues to fill until atrial contraction occurs. Atrial contraction contributes the final volume for ventricular filling.

Pulmonary circulation

The right side of the cardiac pump, consisting of the right atrium and right ventricle, delivers venous blood to the lungs for oxygenation. The thin-walled pulmonary vessels have little medial muscle and offer six times less resistance than systemic blood vessels. Since the pulmonary vessels offer little resistance, the right ventricle is considered a low-pressure pump.

Systemic circulation

The left side of the cardiac pump, consisting of the left atrium and left ventricle, generates the high pressures necessary to overcome peripheral vascular resistance and to deliver oxygenated arterial blood to all body tissues. Because the left ventricle has a larger muscle mass than the right ventricle, must generate more pressure, and contract with greater strength, it has a greater need for oxygen. Thus, the left ventricle is particularly susceptible to the effects of deficient oxygen supply.

Coronary circulation

Coronary artery circulation delivers oxygenated blood to the heart, primarily during diastole. The small coronary arteries branch off the aorta and encircle the heart at the epicardial layer.

The arteries continue to branch and enter the myocardium and endocardium, becoming arterioles and then capillaries. The right coronary artery branches to the right from the aorta and supplies blood to the right atrium, the right ventricle, the sinoatrial (SA) and atrioventricular (AV) nodes of the conduction system, and, in most people, the inferior-posterior wall of the left ventricle. The left coronary artery bifurcates into the left anterior descending and circumflex coronary arteries. The left anterior descending artery supplies part of the left and right ventricles and the interventricular septum. The circumflex artery supplies the left atrium and the lateral wall of the left ventricle. In some people, the circumflex artery also provides oxygenated blood to the posterior surfaces of the left atrium and left ventricle.

Hemodynamics

Cardiac output refers to the volume of blood ejected by the left ventricle into the aorta in 1 minute—normally, about 4 to 6 liters/minute at rest. Cardiac output is a product of the heart rate multiplied by the stroke volume, the amount of blood ejected from the left ventricle with each beat. The heart rate may vary from second to second or minute to minute. The stroke volume may vary from beat to beat.

CORONARY ARTERY CIRCULATION

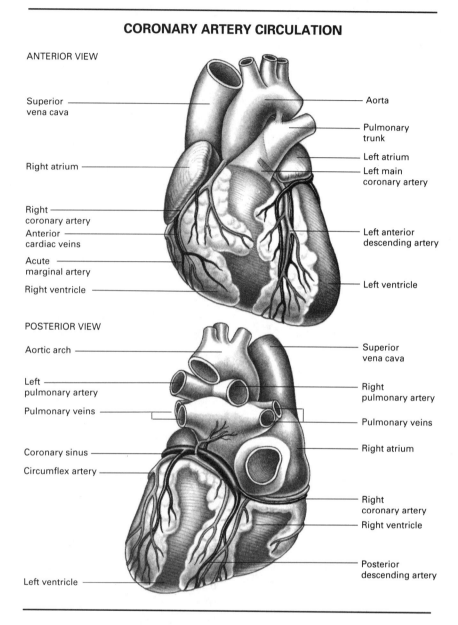

ANTERIOR VIEW

Superior vena cava — Aorta

— Pulmonary trunk

Right atrium —
— Left atrium
— Left main coronary artery

Right coronary artery —
Anterior cardiac veins —
— Left anterior descending artery

Acute marginal artery —
Right ventricle —
— Left ventricle

POSTERIOR VIEW

Aortic arch —
— Superior vena cava

Left pulmonary artery —
— Right pulmonary artery

Pulmonary veins —
— Pulmonary veins

Coronary sinus —
— Right atrium

Circumflex artery —
— Right coronary artery
— Right ventricle

Left ventricle —
— Posterior descending artery

Heart rate

A change in heart rate can dramatically affect cardiac output. For instance, when the heart rate increases, cardiac output may double or triple. In a person with heart disease, such an increase can be dangerous because it decreases diastolic filling time, increases oxygen demand, and decreases coronary artery perfusion time. Conversely, if the heart rate falls below 50 beats/minute, cardiac output usually decreases.

Stroke volume

Variables influencing the stroke volume include preload, afterload, and contractility. *Preload* is the volume of blood that fills the ventricle at the end of diastole. An increase in diastolic volume increases muscle stretch and subsequent stroke volume. Either excessive or inadequate preload can increase the heart's work load and decrease the stroke volume. *Afterload,* the resistance to flow from the ventricle, increases secondary to vasoconstriction in the peripheral blood vessels or to increased resistance, such as aortic stenosis. Increases in afterload result in greater oxygen demand because the heart must use more contractile energy to eject blood. *Contractility* refers to the ability of cardiac muscle fibers to shorten. Calcium within the cell allows protein fibers to be attracted to each other, causing muscle shortening. The contractile (or inotropic) state of the myocardium can be influenced by many factors. For instance, epinephrine, dopamine, and sympathetic nervous system stimulation exert a positive inotropic effect (increase contractility), whereas hypoxemia, acidosis, and such drugs as propranolol (Inderal) exert a negative inotropic effect (decrease contractility).

Arterial blood pressure

The pressure exerted on the arterial wall as blood flows through the arteries is called *arterial blood pressure,* a product of the cardiac output and the *total peripheral resistance,* which is determined by blood viscosity and by the length and internal diameter of the vessels. Arteries have a medial or muscle layer in their wall that permits constriction or dilation of the vessel. Thus, peripheral vascular resistance and blood pressure are affected by vasoconstriction and vasodilation.

Cardiac innervation

Innervation of the heart involves the autonomic nervous system and the baroreceptor and Bainbridge reflexes.

Autonomic nervous system

The autonomic nervous system influences cardiac activity through sympathetic and parasympathetic nerve fibers. Sympathetic fibers are found in the atrial and ventricular walls, the SA and AV nodes. The sympathetic effect on the heart is mediated through beta receptor sites and release of norepinephrine. Stimulation of $beta_1$ receptors increases heart rate, conduction velocity, and contractility. The major effects are usually on the SA node, increasing heart rate, and the myocardial muscle. The sympathetic nervous system also has receptor sites, primarily alpha and $beta_2$ receptors, in peripheral blood vessels. When the sympathetic nervous system is stimulated, the alpha effects predominate in the blood vessels and cause vasoconstriction. The parasympathetic effects on the heart are mediated through release of acetylcholine at nerve endings in the SA node, atrial muscle, and AV node. Parasympathetic or vagal stimulation decreases heart rate and conduction velocity.

Baroreceptor and Bainbridge reflexes

The baroreceptor reflex mediates heart rate as well as peripheral vascular resistance. The baroreceptors—specialized "pressure-sensitive" tissue located in the aortic arch and carotid sinuses—increase their rate of discharge when they are stretched by increased blood pressure. Impulses are transmitted to the cardiovascular center in the medulla. The cardiovascular center decreases sympathetic stimulation and increases parasympathetic stimulation, thereby decreasing heart rate and initiating blood vessel dilation. Conversely, baroreceptors also respond to decreasing blood pressure by increasing heart rate and vasoconstriction.

The Bainbridge reflex is thought to be mediated by stretch receptors in the atria. These receptors may respond to increased volume and cause an increase in heart rate. Contractility is unaffected by the Bainbridge reflex.

Cardiac conduction system

The cardiac conduction system initiates and transmits electrical impulses throughout the heart to achieve the rhythmic beating that makes the heart an efficient pump. This property of self-initiating electrical impulses is called *automaticity*. The property of transmitting electrical impulses from cell to cell along a fiber length is called *conductivity*.

The SA node, also called the sinus node, is the heart's normal pacemaker. Located on the posterior wall of the right atrium near the juncture of the superior vena cava, the SA node normally has a faster rate of automaticity than other areas of the conduction system. Consequently, the SA node assumes dominance as a pacemaker by discharging at a rate faster than any other cardiac site. The normal pacing rate for the sinus node is 60 to 100 beats/minute.

Internodal pathways and Bachmann's bundle conduct electrical impulses through the atria. The internodal pathways converge in the AV node at the base of the right atrium, on the border of the leaflet of the tricuspid valve. The AV node, slow in conducting and slow in recovering, protects the ventricles from fast rates and allows time for ventricular filling. The impulse continues down to the bundle of His, an appendage of the AV node, and into the interventricular septum.

The AV node and the bundle of His together are referred to as the AV junction. Impulses are transmitted faster when they leave the AV node and move into the bundle of His. The AV junction serves as a secondary pacemaker (also called an escape or ectopic pacemaker) if

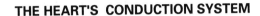

THE HEART'S CONDUCTION SYSTEM

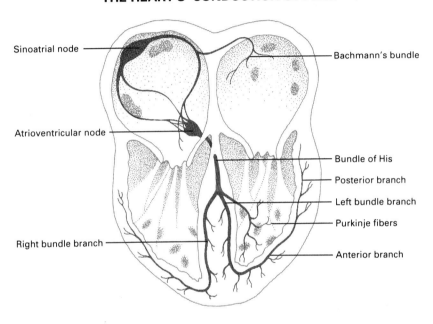

the SA node slows significantly or fails to fire. The normal pacing rate for the AV junction is 40 to 60 beats/minute. The bundle of His bifurcates into the right and left bundle branches. The right bundle branch runs down the right side of the interventricular septum close to the surface. The left bundle branch bifurcates into anterior and posterior fascicles, or branches. Both bundle branches end in a network of Purkinje fibers that completely line the endocardial surface of the ventricular chambers. Like the AV junction, the Purkinje fibers can serve as a secondary pacemaker. The normal pacing rate of the Purkinje fibers is 15 to 40 beats/minute.

2

Electrophysiology and the ECG

An electrical current originates from electrolyte move-

ment across cell membranes. As one cell stimulates

another, the current is recorded and measured by an

electrocardiogram (ECG). This chapter explores elec-

trophysiologic activity and explains methods of mea-

suring and comparing resultant ECG waveforms to

obtain useful diagnostic information.

Electrophysiology of the cardiac cycle

Cells of the conduction system and of the myocardium have properties that permit depolarization (producing contraction) and repolarization (producing relaxation) in response to electrolyte movements
across the cell membrane. Normally, extracellular fluid has a higher
concentration of sodium ions, and intracellular fluid has a higher
concentration of potassium ions. A myocardial cell at rest or in a
polarized state has a transmembrane action potential of -90 millivolts
(mV). An action potential is a rapid change in electrical activity
caused by ion diffusion at the cell membrane. The inside of the cell
is negatively charged; the outside, positively charged.

Depolarization begins with an extracellular stimulus from one cell
to another and continues along a fiber length. During depolarization,
fast-sodium channels are open, bringing a rapid influx of sodium.
Because sodium carries a positive charge, the inside of the cell
membrane becomes less negatively charged. A transmembrane
action potential is recorded by measuring this process at the cell
membrane.

MYOCARDIAL TRANSMEMBRANE ACTION POTENTIAL

This schematic representation depicts ventricular myocardial working cell action potential. Arrows
indicate major ionic movement across the cell membrane.

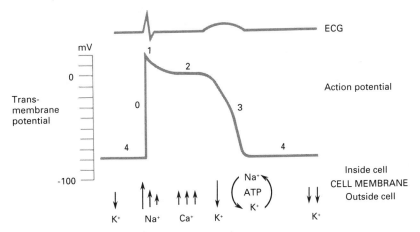

Adapted with permission from Textbook of Advanced Cardiac Life Support, *2nd ed., 1987. Copyright American Heart Association.*

Once a threshold level is reached, the action potential automatically continues. The threshold is the point at which a stimulus causes
excitation of a fiber. During depolarization, the rapid influx of sodium
creates a sudden upswing (phase 0) followed by a peak and slight

drop (phase 1). The less negative potential allows for opening of the slow calcium-sodium channels, facilitating an influx of calcium and sodium. The increasing intracellular concentration of calcium causes an efflux of potassium via potassium channels (phase 2). The outflow of potassium triggers active repolarization (phase 3) and eventual muscle relaxation by initiating active transport of sodium and potassium across the cell membrane. This active pumping is fueled by adenosine triphosphate (ATP). Once electrolyte concentrations return to normal across the membrane, the resting potential is reached (phase 4), the process is complete, and the polarized cell is ready to be restimulated.

Cells of the conduction system, particularly the sinoatrial (SA) node, the atrioventricular (AV) node, and the Purkinje fibers, have the property of automaticity; that is, the cells can depolarize spontaneously without an extracellular stimulus to the cell membrane. Automaticity occurs because of the difference in the resting potential (phase 4) of these conduction system cells.

PACEMAKER CELL ACTION POTENTIAL

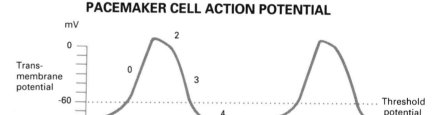

Reprinted with permission from Textbook of Advanced Cardiac Life Support, *2nd ed., 1987. Copyright American Heart Association.*

The resting potential is approximately -55 to -65 mV. At this potential, the slow channels open, allowing for the slow influx of calcium and sodium, which causes depolarization. Once again potassium drifts out through the potassium channels, triggering active repolarization via the potassium-sodium pump. As the resting potential is reached, ions immediately leak back into the cell; when the threshold level is reached, another impulse is discharged. This leak of ions creates the automaticity, or automatic pacing rate, of pacemaker cells in the conduction system.

From the time depolarization begins until the repolarization phase is well under way, the cell cannot respond again. This property is called refractoriness. During phases 0, 1, and 2, the cell is absolutely refractory; even a strong stimulus will not elicit a response. The cell then enters a relative refractory period (phase 3) in which a response may or may not be elicited. A vulnerable period occurs toward the end of phase 3, during which the stimulus might elicit a repetitive or chaotic response.

Basics of electrocardiography

When electrical activity is transmitted from one cell to the next along a fiber length, a current develops. This electrical current is transmitted to the body surface and may be recorded and measured by a surface ECG. The ECG uses a positive (+) and a negative (-) electrode to create a lead (or reference) line for recording electrical activity. When the electrical current travels along the lead line or parallel to it, the lead records the current. An upward deflection indicates a positive current; that is, one traveling toward the positive electrode and away from the negative electrode. A downward deflection indicates a negative current; that is, one traveling toward the negative electrode and away from the positive electrode. Lack of a current or a current perpendicular to the lead line causes an isoelectric (flat) baseline.

A normal cardiac cycle recorded on an ECG produces a series of waves, as an electrical impulse travels from the SA node, through the atria, AV junction, bundle branches, and Purkinje fibers, and out to the myocardium. The normal wave sequence is P-QRS-T, the waves corresponding to the phases of the action potential. The sequence repeats with each cardiac cycle.

The P wave, the first wave of the cardiac cycle, represents depolarization of the atria. In most leads the P wave is small, rounded, and upright (positive), but in some leads it may be inverted (negative) or biphasic (above and below the baseline). A return to the baseline marks the end of the P wave, as the electrical impulse slows in the AV node and moves through the bundle of His.

The QRS complex, a series of vectors or directions of current representing depolarization of the ventricles, begins when the electrical impulse reaches the bundle branches. The first wave in the complex, the Q wave, is negative and has a downward deflection. The R wave that follows is positive, with an upward deflection. The next wave, the S wave, is negative. A second R wave in a QRS complex, called an R prime, sometimes occurs. Uppercase or lowercase letters designate the voltage or height of one wave as compared to another in the QRS complex. Note also that not all QRS complexes contain all three waves.

MYOCARDIAL ACTION POTENTIAL CURVE

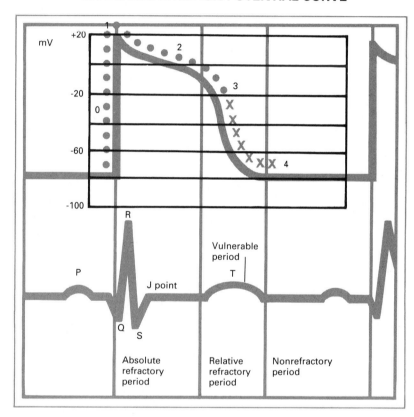

CONFIGURATIONS OF QRS COMPLEXES

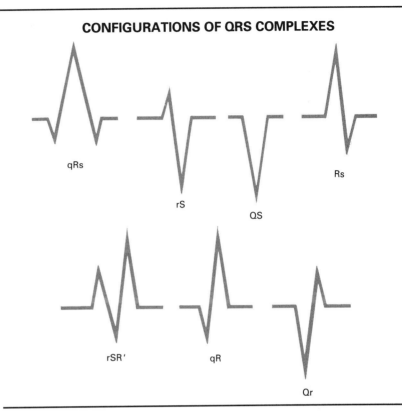

Of all cardiac impulses, the QRS complex usually has the largest voltage and thus the tallest waves. The QRS complex ends with the start of the ST segment, which is usually isoelectric in the normal heart. The angle at which the QRS complex ends and the ST segment begins is called the J point. If the ST segment is elevated or depressed, the J point will deviate from the isoelectric line.

J POINT

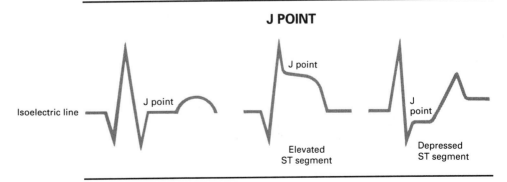

The ST segment corresponds to the plateau phase (phase 2) of the transmembrane action potential and is followed by the T wave, which represents ventricular repolarization. T waves are usually rounded and of lower voltage than the QRS complex. Like P waves, T waves may be upright, inverted, or biphasic. U waves sometimes occur in the cardiac cycle. The U wave follows the T wave, is of a lower voltage, and is related to a delay in movement of potassium across the cell membrane. The U wave occurs in patients with hypokalemia or with high blood levels of quinidine.

ECG measurements

The ECG tracing is recorded on graph paper consisting of 1-mm squares:

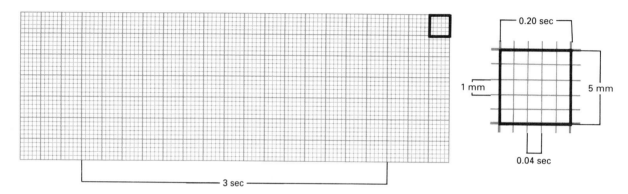

An ECG recorder moves the paper under the recording stylus at a speed of 25 mm/second. Thus, the duration of waves and the distance between waves can be measured to determine heart rates and conduction intervals.

Calculating heart rates

You can use one of two methods to calculate an approximate heart rate. Refer to the illustration below and to the bulleted instructions that follow.

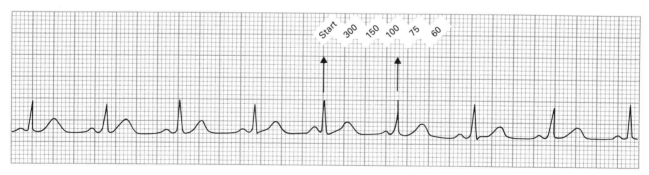

• Obtain a 6-second ECG strip by counting 30 large boxes on the graphed ECG paper across the recording or by using the 1-second or 3-second markings on the ECG paper. Multiply the number of QRS complexes in the 6-second strip by 10. Using this method for the example above, you would determine a heart rate of about 90 beats/ minute (9 QRS complexes multiplied by 10).

• If the rhythm is essentially regular (no more than 0.04 second or one small box variation from R to R), you can use another method. Since the paper moves at a speed of 25 mm/second, the stylus covers 300 large (5-mm) boxes per minute. Count the number of large boxes between QRS complexes and divide 300 by this number to determine the heart rate. Using this method for the example above, you would determine a heart rate of about 86 beats/minute (300 divided by 3.5 large boxes).

Measuring conduction intervals

To determine conduction intervals and recognize signs of AV blocks, measure the PR interval—the distance from the beginning of the P wave to the beginning of the QRS complex. This distance represents the time the impulse travels from the SA node through the atria and AV junction to the bundle branches. The normal PR interval is 0.12 to 0.20 second (3 to 5 small boxes on the ECG paper).

The QRS complex duration is measured from the beginning of the QRS complex as it leaves the baseline (regardless of whether it starts with a Q or an R wave) to the point at which it angles off to the ST segment (the J point). The normal QRS complex duration is less than 0.12 second (fewer than 3 small boxes on the ECG paper). A longer QRS complex indicates a delay in interventricular conduction.

ECG lead placement

A standard ECG is recorded in 12 different leads to obtain a complete picture of cardiac electrical activity. The 12-lead ECG allows a view of electrical activity on two planes, frontal and horizontal (transverse). Ten electrodes are placed on the patient: two on the arms, two on the legs, and six on the chest. The right leg electrode is always used as a reference (or ground) electrode. The other electrodes are designated as negative or positive in any given lead as recording is taking place.

The first six leads look at the frontal plane of the heart, and the first three of these are bipolar leads, with each lead making use of one positive and one negative electrode. In lead I, the positive electrode is on the left arm, and the negative electrode is on the right arm. This view records current moving toward the left side of the body as a positive wave.

In lead II, the positive electrode is on the left leg, and the negative electrode is on the right arm. Thus, current traveling down and to the left will be recorded as upward, or positive, deflections. This lead follows the long axis of the heart and, in most people, tends to produce the tallest, most positive waves.

In lead III, the positive electrode is on the left leg, and the negative electrode is on the left arm. Leads I, II, and III form a triangle around the heart known as Einthoven's triangle.

EINTHOVEN'S TRIANGLE

Standard limb leads

The next three leads—aV_R, aV_L, and aV_F—are augmented voltage leads. The last letter in the name of each lead designates the unipolar positive lead placement, and the negative is represented by the ECG machine, using a combination of the other electrodes. In aV_R, the right arm electrode is positive, and the negative is down and to the left. In aV_L, the left arm electrode is positive, and the negative is down and to the right. In aV_F, the positive electrode is on the left leg (foot), and the negative is straight up through the center of the body.

Thus, the first six leads view electrical activity on the frontal plane of the heart, measuring current that travels superior, inferior, left, or right.

FRONTAL PLANE OF THE HEART AS VIEWED
BY LIMB LEADS

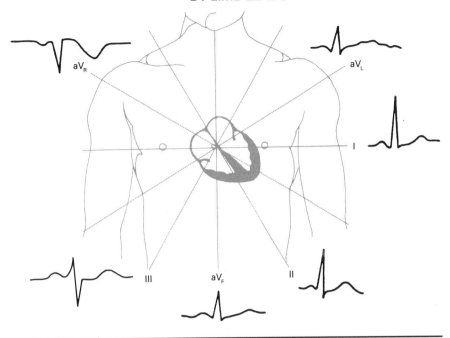

The remaining six leads of the 12-lead ECG are the chest (precordial) leads, V_1 to V_6, which view the horizontal plane.

HORIZONTAL PLANE OF THE HEART AS VIEWED
BY CHEST LEADS

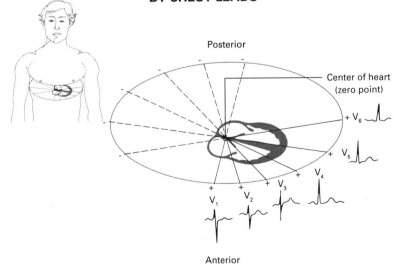

In each of the unipolar chest leads, the chest electrode is positive, and the ECG combines the three limb electrodes (right arm, left arm, and left leg) to provide the negative end of the lead. The negative thus becomes the center of the body, permitting measurement of current from anterior, posterior, lateral left, and lateral right views of the heart to create the horizontal plane.

One-lead recording is commonly used for monitoring a patient during transport to a hospital or in an emergency room or critical care unit. To allow the patient more freedom of movement, electrodes are moved from the limbs to the chest. The two most common leads used for monitoring are lead II and the modified chest lead, MCL_1.

In lead II monitoring, the right arm electrode is moved to the right shoulder, and the left leg electrode is moved to the lower left chest. In MCL_1 monitoring, the positive electrode is placed at the fourth intercostal space to the right of the sternum (V_1 position), and the negative electrode is placed on the left shoulder.

ELECTRODE PLACEMENT FOR CHEST LEADS

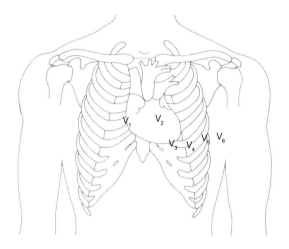

- V_1—fourth intercostal space at the right border of the sternum

- V_2—fourth intercostal space at the left border of the sternum

- V_3—halfway between V_2 and V_4

- V_4—fifth intercostal space at the midclavicular line

- V_5—anterior axillary line (halfway between V_4 and V_6)

- V_6—midaxillary line, level with V_4

ECG MONITORING ELECTRODE PLACEMENT

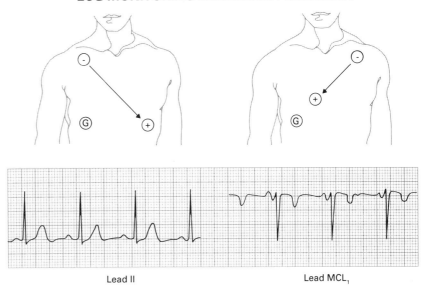

Lead II	Lead MCL₁

The recording obtained in MCL$_1$ mimics a V$_1$ recording and, therefore, usually has a biphasic P wave (above and below the isoelectric line) and a negative QRS complex— commonly an rS wave. This lead is helpful in determining aberrantly conducted beats and positions the electrodes out of the way if defibrillator paddle placement is necessary.

A recording from a single-lead ECG monitoring system may be used to determine cardiac rate and rhythm. However, a 12-lead ECG should be used to obtain additional diagnostic information (see Chapter 3, The 12-Lead ECG).

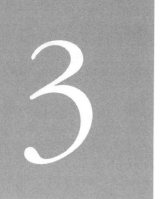

The 12-Lead ECG

The 12-lead electrocardiogram (ECG) provides a two-dimensional view of cardiac electrical activity, with each lead revealing information about a particular segment of that activity or presenting information about the heart from a different vantage point. By comparing information obtained from different leads, you can develop a more comprehensive picture of electrical activity— and thus a more accurate picture of the patient's clinical status.

Axis

The first six leads of the normal 12-lead ECG encircle the heart on the frontal plane, each lead viewing the heart from the vantage point of the positive electrode looking toward the negative electrode. Either a positive or negative end of a lead is situated every 30 degrees around the circle, with each lead looking directly across the heart.

HEXAXIAL REFERENCE CIRCLE

As these illustrations show, moving the three sides of Einthoven's triangle along parallel positions until they intersect in the middle of the heart (1) and then superimposing the three augmented voltage leads as each intersects in the middle of the heart (2) produces the hexaxial reference circle (3). The circle is used to determine the electrical axis of the heart in the frontal plane.

1.

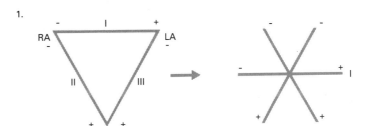

2.

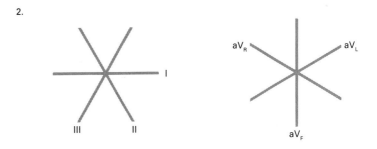

3.

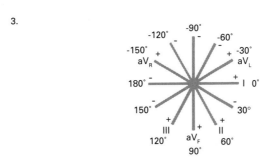

In the normal heart, the interventricular septum is the first part of the ventricles activated by an electrical current. This activation is from left to right, providing an initial vector, or direction of current, toward the right ventricle. The current then travels through the bundle branches and stimulates the apex of both ventricles, which provides the next vector. This stimulation is followed by complete activation of the right ventricle. Activation of the left ventricle overlaps activation of the right, so the vectors somewhat balance each other. However, because the left ventricle has a larger muscle mass, the wave of depolarization takes longer on the left side, which shifts the vector up and to the left.

SEQUENCE OF VENTRICULAR ACTIVATION

The illustrations below reveal the sequence of ventricular activation in a normal heart: the septal vector (1), as the electrical impulse activates the interventricular septum from left to right; the apical vector (2), as the impulse travels through both bundle branches toward the apices; activation of both ventricles (3), as the impulse spreads throughout the ventricular walls; and activation of the remainder of the left ventricle (4), as the impulse travels through its larger muscle mass. Arrows represent the direction and magnitude of the heart's electrical current.

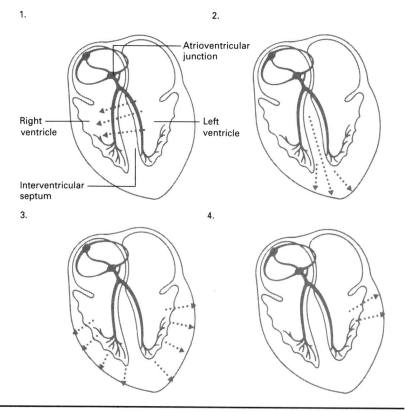

The mean QRS vector, the sum of the heart's small vectors, represents the axis, or general direction of ventricular depolarization. A normal axis on the frontal plane points downward and to the patient's left side, between 0 and 90 degrees on the hexaxial reference circle. Thus, in a normal heart, the tallest, most positive QRS complex would be found in one of the leads with its positive end between 0 and 90 degrees on this circle: I, II, or aV$_F$. Any negative wave in the QRS complex is subtracted from the height of the R wave. For instance, if lead II has an R wave 10 mm tall and an S wave 2 mm deep, the height of the QRS complex is 8 mm. Another QRS complex may have only an R wave, 9 mm tall, without a negative wave (Q or S) and would therefore be the tallest, most positive complex.

An abnormality in the heart causes the vector to shift or deviate. If the tallest, most positive QRS complex is found in lead III, then the axis has shifted down and to the right, indicating right axis deviation (RAD). If lead aV$_L$ is the most positive, then the axis has shifted up and to the left, indicating left axis deviation (LAD). Common causes of RAD include right ventricular hypertrophy, left posterior hemiblock, and lateral wall myocardial infarction (MI). Common causes of LAD include left ventricular hypertrophy, left anterior hemiblock, and inferior-posterior MI.

AXIS DEVIATION

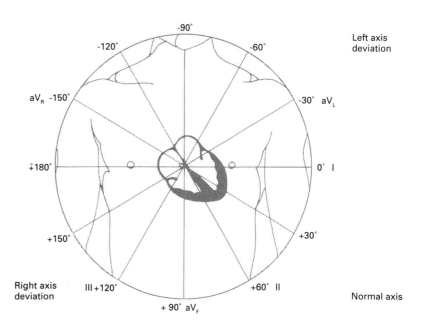

Ischemia, injury, and infarction

When coronary circulation is diminished or blocked, the myocardium undergoes a dynamic series of changes. These changes are reflected by alterations in 12-lead ECG recordings, which provide information about the type and location of damage.

As mentioned in Chapter 2, the ST segment represents the plateau phase of the action potential, during which an influx of calcium and an efflux of potassium occur. The T wave represents active repolarization via potassium-sodium pumps. Both processes require adequate oxygen delivery to the cell. Ischemia or inadequate oxygen supply will affect these two phases of electrical activity and thus alter the ECG recording.

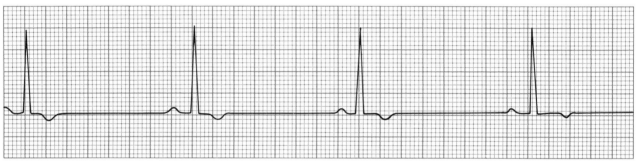

Ischemia: Inverted T wave.

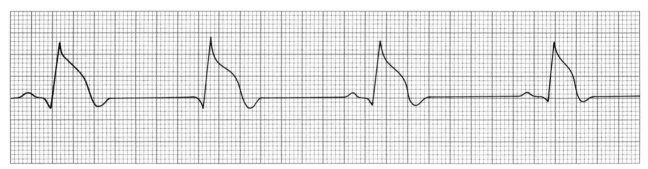

Injury: Elevated ST segment.

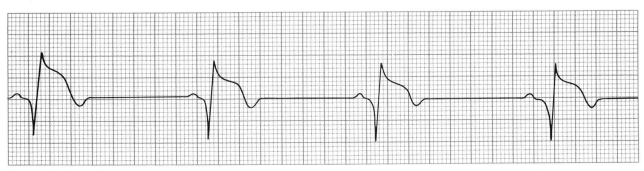

Necrosis: Pathologic Q wave.

As shown in the ECG strips above, ischemia is represented by an inverted T wave in the leads in which the positive electrode reads across the ischemic myocardium. Injury is represented by ST segment elevation in the leads in which the positive electrode reads across the injured or severely ischemic myocardium. In an MI, myocardial tissue necroses. This necrosed tissue no longer has the electrophysiologic properties of a normal myocardium. The infarcted area does not depolarize or repolarize and eventually fills with scar tissue. A lead reading across this area records the vector on the opposite normal wall, unopposed by vectors from the infarcted wall of the ventricle. The lead would record the vectors as traveling away from the positive electrode and would show a Q wave. A Q wave that is at least a quarter the height of the R wave usually indicates MI (although conduction delays, such as bundle branch blocks, can also cause Q waves).

Thus, ST segment and T wave changes and pathologic Q waves can indicate ischemia, injury, and infarction, and you can use the leads that record these changes to identify the location of the abnormality:

II, III, aV_F — inferior
I, aV_L, V_1, V_2, V_3 — anteroseptal
I, aV_L, V_5, V_6 — anterolateral
I, aV_L, V_4 — anteroapical
V_1, V_2 (reciprocal changes) — posterior

Acute inferior MI

To examine further how ECG changes help identify the type and location of myocardial damage, review the following ECG strips. The first one shows early changes of an inferior-wall MI:

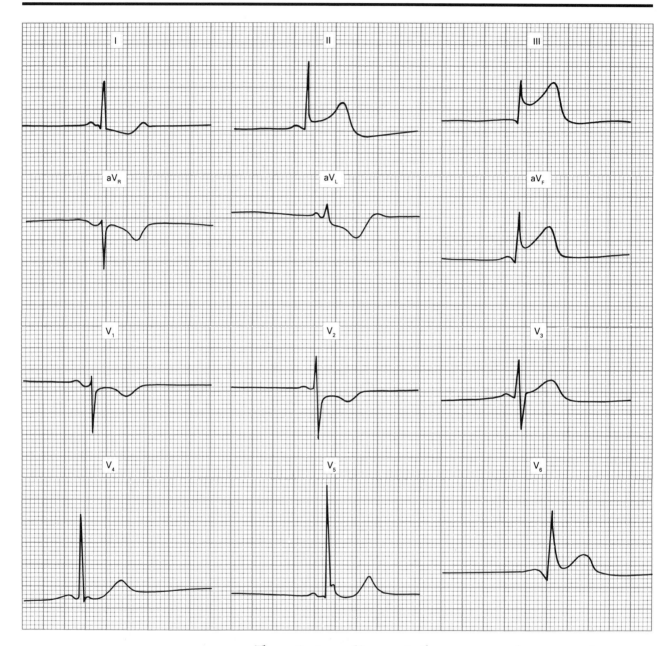

The patient, age 59, came to the emergency department after having chest pain for 10 hours. He was pale and diaphoretic. His blood pressure was 92/50 mm Hg; pulse rate, 48 beats/minute; respiratory rate, 26 breaths/minute. The first ECG taken in the emergency department shows early changes of acute injury (ST segment elevations in leads II, III, and aV_F) and reciprocal changes (depressed ST segments in leads I and aV_L). Initially, the hyperacute T wave is accentuated by the elevated ST segment; as the patient's condition evolves, the T wave will invert and the Q wave will develop. This ECG shows just a slight Q wave in the inferior leads. The patient also has a sinus bradycardia. Bradycardias and atrioventricular (AV) blocks are common complications associated with inferior-wall MIs and may need emergency treatment.

The next strip is from the same patient 48 hours after admission:

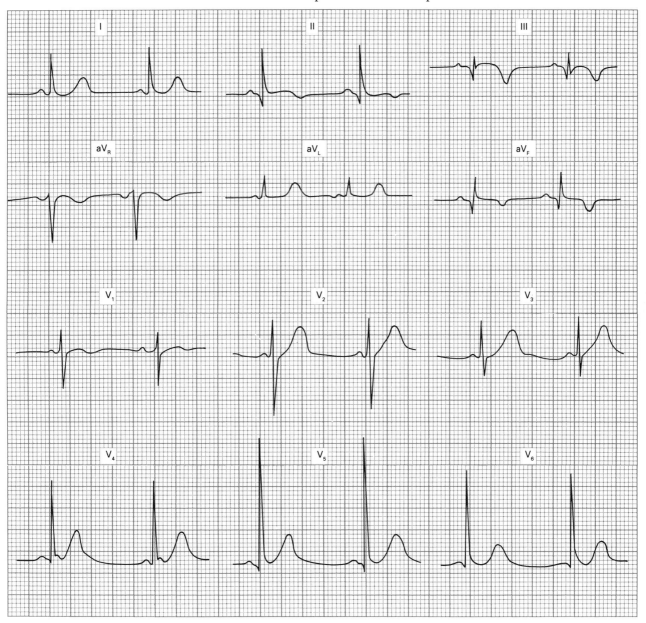

This recording shows well-developed Q waves in leads II, III, and aV_F. The ST segments have returned to baseline, and the T waves have inverted. ST segment and T wave changes are reversible, but the Q wave commonly remains as a permanent addition to the ECG. Thus, Q waves without the acute changes of ST segment elevation and T wave inversion may signal a previous MI. Some infarctions are intramural; they do not fully extend through the ventricular wall. An intramural infarction may produce ST and T wave changes without the typical Q waves. Diagnosis of these infarctions depends on the patient's signs and symptoms and on results of cardiac enzyme studies.

Reciprocal changes

When ischemia, injury, or infarction occurs, the lead reading across the damaged area records the positive or pathologic changes; the lead on the opposite side records reciprocal changes, which appear as mirror images of the changes caused by ischemia, injury, or infarction. Thus, an elevated ST segment in the affected lead will appear as a depressed ST segment in a lead reading from the opposite side of the heart. In an acute inferior-wall MI, Q waves, ST segment elevation, and inverted T waves may occur in leads II, III, and aV_F, and reciprocal changes — tall R waves, ST segment depression, and upright T waves — will occur in leads I and aV_L. In a wall of the heart that does not have a lead reading across it, damage may be diagnosed by viewing reciprocal changes in a lead reading from the opposite side. An example of this would be the posterior wall of the left ventricle, which has no positive electrode reading from the posterior toward the anterior of the body. However, because leads V_1 and V_2 read from anterior to posterior, reciprocal changes in V_1 and V_2 would indicate posterior MI.

The standard 12-lead ECG does not directly read right ventricular activity. If a right ventricular infarction is suspected (because of inferior-posterior wall MI and a clinical picture of right ventricular failure), then additional electrodes — V_3R, V_4R, V_5R, and V_6R — may be applied. Positive changes of ischemia, injury, or infarction are then discerned from these leads.

ELECTRODE PLACEMENT FOR RIGHT VENTRICULAR INFARCTION

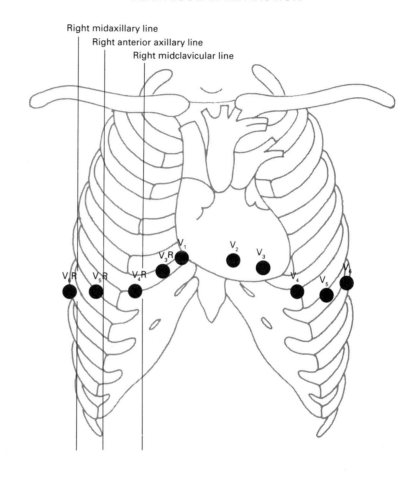

The effectiveness of initial therapy for an MI can also be observed on the ECG. Reperfusion with vasodilators and thrombolytic agents is becoming more common in the early hours after onset of symptoms. Reversal of ST elevation and T wave inversion will show on the ECG as reperfusion occurs. The same effect may be seen in some patients with a percutaneous transluminal angioplasty or balloon catheter dilation of a stenosed coronary artery.

Interventricular conduction delays

Interventricular conduction delays are caused by complete or partial blocking of an electrical impulse in an area of the bundle branch–Purkinje conduction system. This delay causes an abnormal widening of the QRS complex.

Conduction blocks

A bundle branch block can occur in either the right or left fascicles of the conduction system. A right bundle branch block (RBBB) occurs when conduction is blocked in the right bundle branch while the impulse travels normally through the left bundle branch. Usually, the septum is activated normally, with a delay in right ventricular activation as the impulse travels across the septum from the left bundle branch and finally activates the right ventricle in a fiber-to-fiber manner.

ACTIVATION OF THE VENTRICLES IN RIGHT BUNDLE BRANCH BLOCK

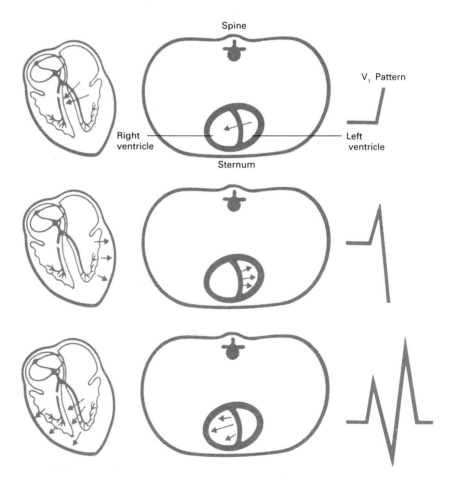

This altered conduction prolongs the QRS complex to 0.12 second or greater and changes the normal shape of the QRS complex, frequently causing a triphasic pattern or an abnormally prolonged or distorted R wave in leads V_1 or MCL_1.

RIGHT BUNDLE BRANCH BLOCK PATTERNS

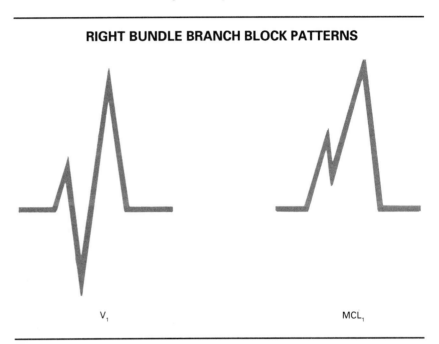

V_1 MCL_1

Thus, in these leads, the RBBB is characterized by distortion of the terminal R wave. These widened complexes occur whenever an impulse originates above the ventricle.

A left bundle branch block (LBBB) occurs when conduction is blocked either in the left bundle branch before it bifurcates or in both the anterior and posterior fascicles of the left conduction system. LBBB is typified by a widened QRS complex (0.12 second or greater) and, in lead V_1 or MCL_1, a widened, notched QS complex or an rS complex with a widened, distorted S wave. Note that both RBBB and LBBB also produce altered T waves.

LEFT BUNDLE BRANCH BLOCK PATTERNS

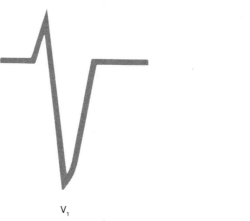

V₁

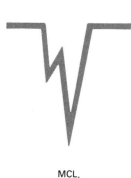

MCL₁

Hemiblocks — conduction blocks in either the left anterior or left posterior fascicles — do not usually widen the QRS complex. Hemiblocks may be diagnosed by information obtained from several leads. ECG criteria for a left anterior hemiblock include LAD, a small Q wave in leads I and aV$_L$, and a small R wave in lead III. Criteria for a left posterior hemiblock include RAD, a small Q wave in lead III, and a small R wave in leads I and aV$_L$.

You can evaluate the possibility of an RBBB progressing to complete heart block by looking for a hemiblock. A bifascicular block, particularly the combination of an RBBB and a left posterior hemiblock, appears more likely to progress to complete heart block if it develops during an acute MI. Because these two fascicles are anatomically isolated from each other, injury to both conduction pathways usually indicates widespread damage. A pacemaker may be inserted prophylactically for this type of bifascicular block, particularly if it occurs with a first- or second-degree AV block.

Aberrations

A patient may experience an isolated ectopic or supraventricular tachycardia, with a widened, distorted QRS complex, although the patient's underlying rhythm is normal, with otherwise normal QRS complexes. The isolated abnormal QRS complex is aberrantly conducted; that is, the impulse takes an abnormal or aberrant pathway through the ventricles. The aberration is usually caused by a premature impulse traveling through the conduction system and arriving at the bundle branch at a time when it is partially or totally refractory. The impulse then becomes blocked or delayed, creating an abnormal vector and a widened QRS complex. Because the right bundle branch is normally the last part of the conduction system to repolarize, the aberration usually looks like the pattern characteristic of an RBBB.

Aberrantly conducted impulses are important to identify because they can look similar to premature ventricular contractions or ventricular tachycardia. Note that using the shape of the QRS complex as a distinguishing criterion necessitates V_1 or MCL_1 monitoring.

DISTINGUISHING SUPRAVENTRICULAR ECTOPY WITH ABERRATION FROM VENTRICULAR ECTOPY

The following chart highlights ECG criteria used to distinguish supraventricular ectopy with aberration from ventricular ectopy. No single criterion should be used to rule out one condition or the other.

Supraventricular ectopy with aberration	Ventricular ectopy
Premature P wave associated with QRS complexes	P waves, if present, are dissociated from the QRS complex
Triphasic RSR' pattern in V_1 or MCL_1	Monophasic or biphasic QRS complex
QRS complex duration usually not longer than 0.14 second	QRS complex duration may exceed 0.14 second
Ashman's phenomenon (wide QRS complex ends a short cycle preceded by a long R-R interval)	Capture beats (a sinus P wave interrupts the tachycardia and conducts a QRS complex)
Right axis deviation with tachycardia	Left axis deviation with tachycardia
	Precordial concordance (precordial lead QRS complexes are either all upright or all negative)

Preexcitation syndromes

A slightly widened, distorted QRS complex may also result when an electrical impulse is conducted through a congenital accessory pathway that parallels the AV junction. The most common accessory pathway, the Kent bundle, is usually located around one of the AV valve rings. Because the Kent bundle does not have the usual conduction delay associated with the AV node, impulses travel more rapidly through it than through the AV node. Early stimulation of the ventricle results in preexcitation of the myocardium—a slow, premature, fiber-to-fiber depolarization characterized by a delta wave or initial slurring to the QRS complex. Conduction through the Kent bundle produces Wolff-Parkinson-White (WPW) syndrome. The remainder of the QRS complex usually reflects normal conduction through the AV node–bundle of His–Purkinje system.

PREEXCITATION OF VENTRICLES THROUGH THE KENT BUNDLE

Conduction of electrical impulses through the Kent bundle results in Wolff-Parkinson-White syndrome. ECG characteristics include a short PR interval and a delta wave that slightly widens the QRS complex, although usually not above 0.12 second. A delta wave is apparent in leads throughout the 12-lead ECG but may appear as a Q wave in some leads, thus mimicking the pattern of a myocardial infarction. The abnormal depolarization may also cause abnormal repolarization, which would be reflected in abnormal T waves.

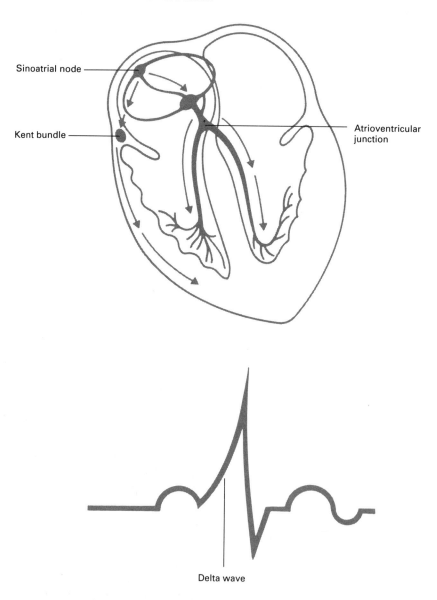

Sinoatrial node

Kent bundle

Atrioventricular junction

Delta wave

WPW syndrome is characterized not only by preexcitation of the ventricles but also by episodes of paroxysmal supraventricular tachycardia caused by a reentry cycle. Reentry cycles may start with one premature atrial depolarization. WPW syndrome carries an increased risk of rapid ventricular response to atrial fibrillation or flutter. Consequently, atrial arrhythmias in a patient with this syndrome usually warrant early intervention with drug therapy.

REENTRY TACHYCARDIA WITH WOLFF-PARKINSON-WHITE SYNDROME

The reentry cycle occurs when a premature impulse travels down the atrioventricular (AV) junction and up the Kent bundle to reenter the atrium or, conversely, down the Kent bundle and back up to the atrium through the AV junction. In the first type of conduction, the QRS remains normal because the impulse is initially conducted through the AV junction. A delta wave is usually associated with the second type of conduction.

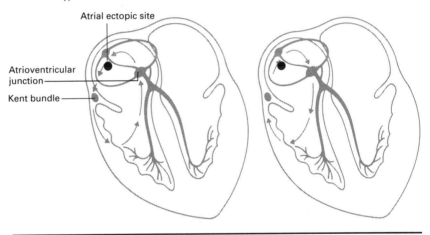

The ECG strip on the next page shows evidence of a wide complex supraventricular tachycardia in a patient with a history of WPW:

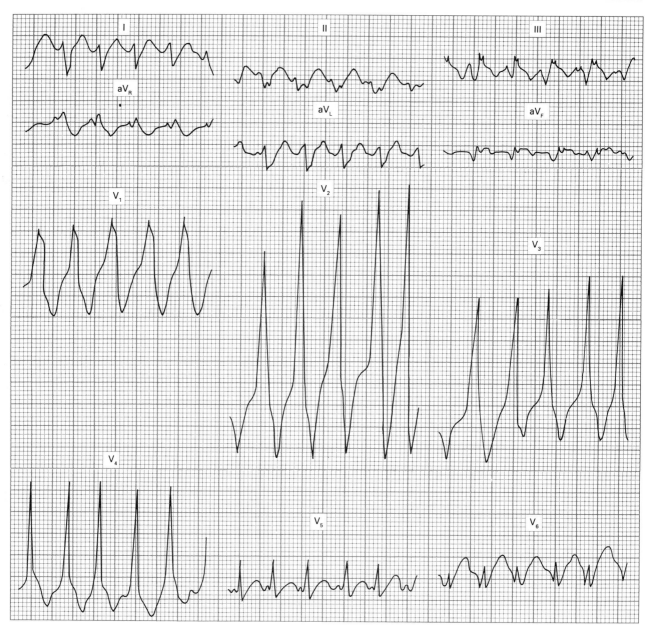

The patient, a 30-year-old male, came to the emergency department complaining of palpitations and light-headedness. Initially, he was treated with procainamide (Pronestyl), but the antiarrhythmic had no effect. The staff then instituted cardioversion, which resulted in a sinus rhythm with the characteristic ECG findings of WPW syndrome:

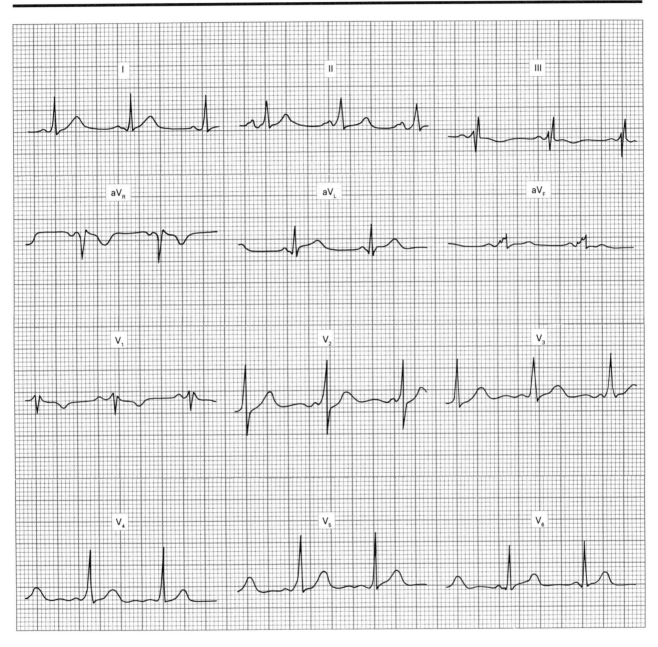

Drug and electrolyte effects

Various drugs and alterations in electrolyte levels can affect cellular electrophysiology. For instance, digoxin (Lanoxin) in a therapeutic dose may cause a downward cove, or recession, of the ST segment that mimics ST segment depression. Digoxin toxicity may produce numerous arrhythmias, including bradycardias, AV blocks, ventricular ectopy, atrial fibrillation, and atrial flutter.

At high blood levels, Class 1A antiarrhythmic agents, such as quinidine sulfate (Quinidex) and procainamide, can affect the ECG. The most common effects are a widened QRS complex and a lengthened QT interval. Widening of the QRS complex by 50% or more is a sign of toxicity. Class II antiarrhythmic agents (beta blockers) may widen the PR interval, and Class IV agents (calcium channel blockers) may slow conduction and lengthen the QT interval.

Abnormal serum potassium levels also affect the ECG. Hyperkalemia widens the QRS complex; produces tall, peaked or tented T waves; alters repolarization; and eventually slows the heart rate. Acute hyperkalemia may produce ventricular fibrillation. Hypokalemia affects cell membrane competency, may produce premature ventricular complexes, enhances the toxic effects of digoxin, and causes short or flattened T waves and U waves.

Arrhythmia Interpretation

This chapter reviews arrhythmia interpretation and implications for clinical intervention. Based on the major electrocardiogram (ECG) criteria for distinguishing each rhythm, the review focuses on wave sequences (as illustrated by the letters P-QRS-T) that will help you identify these criteria.

Rhythms originating in the sinus node

Major rhythms associated with the sinus node include sinus rhythm, sinus bradycardia, sinus tachycardia, sinus arrest, and sinoatrial (SA) block.

Sinus rhythm

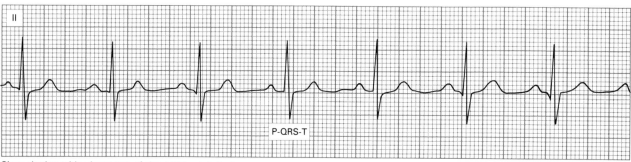

Sinus rhythm with a heart rate of about 72 beats/minute.

Sinus rhythm is the heart's normal rhythm, with a rate of 60 to 100 beats/minute and a normal sequence of P-QRS-T as the impulse follows the normal conduction pathway through the heart. Sinus rhythm is essentially regular; the rate may vary slightly from one heartbeat to the next, but a difference of no more than 0.04 second would be expected in pairs of adjacent beats.

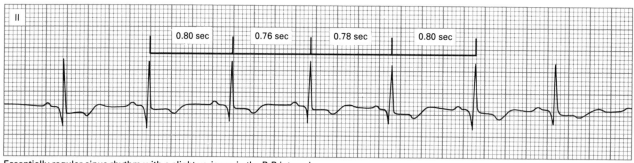

Essentially regular sinus rhythm with a slight variance in the R-R interval.

In lead II, the P wave is upright, but it may be biphasic or inverted in other leads. The same is true of the T wave.

Sinus bradycardia

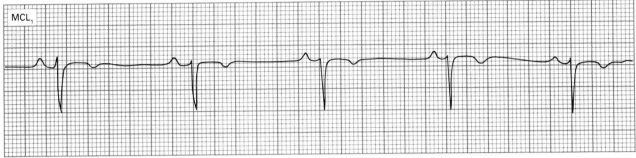

Sinus bradycardia with a heart rate of 48 beats/minute.

Sinus bradycardia has the same wave sequence as sinus rhythm, but the heart rate is less than 60 beats/minute. If the rate decreases below 50 beats/minute, cardiac output usually diminishes, which may lead to dizziness, syncope, premature ventricular ectopy, pallor, chest pain, and hypotension. Symptomatic sinus bradycardia may be caused by an increased vagal effect on the sinus node, drugs, sinus node disease, or ischemia.

Sinus tachycardia

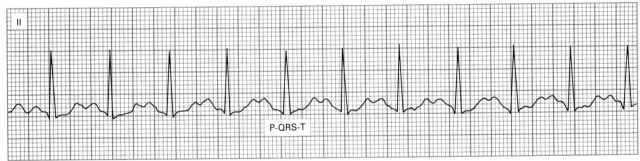

Sinus tachycardia with a heart rate of 110 beats/minute.

Sinus tachycardia is marked by an increase in the firing rate, or automaticity, of the sinus node. The rhythm has a normal wave sequence, but the heart rate is usually between 100 and 160 beats/minute (slightly faster with strenuous exercise). Sinus tachycardia is usually a compensatory response to some underlying physiologic cause, such as exercise, stress, pain, exertion, use of stimulants, or a decrease in blood pressure or cardiac output. Treatment depends on the underlying cause.

Sinus arrest and SA block

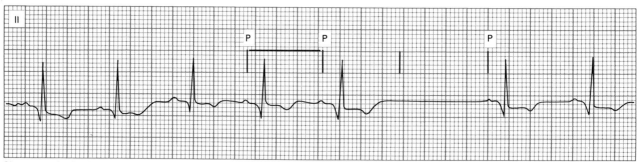

Sinus arrest is characterized by a P-P interval that does not plot across the pause.

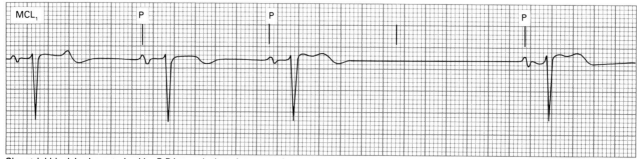

Sinoatrial block is characterized by P-P intervals that plot across the pause.

In sinus arrest and SA block, one or more complete P-QRS-T sequences is missing, thus causing an irregular rhythm. With an underlying sinus rhythm, the wave sequences before and after the pause are usually regular. You can distinguish between sinus arrest and SA block by measuring the interval between the P waves and plotting this interval across the pause. If the interval plots regularly across the pause to the next P wave, the problem is an SA block; if not, it is a sinus arrest. A patient with frequent episodes of sinus arrest or SA block may require treatment for significantly decreased cardiac output.

Rhythms originating in the atria

Major rhythms associated with the atria include premature atrial complex, atrial tachycardia, atrial flutter, and atrial fibrillation.

Premature atrial complex

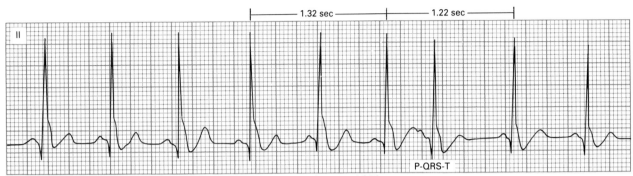

Sinus rhythm with a premature atrial complex (PAC). The distance from the normal QRS complex before the PAC to the normal QRS complex after the PAC is shorter than two normal cycles, indicating a noncompensatory pause.

A premature atrial complex (PAC) is characterized by the appearance of an early P-QRS-T sequence that disturbs the heart's regular rhythm. This early sequence is usually followed by a short pause before the regularity of the dominant rhythm resumes. The P wave of the early sequence may have a different configuration and PR interval than those of the normal rhythm because it originates outside the SA node and follows a different pathway. However, the PR interval should be at least 0.12 second.

Occasionally, the PAC occurs so early that the atrioventricular (AV) node is refractory and cannot transmit conduction to the ventricle. In this instance, the PAC becomes blocked, or nonconducted:

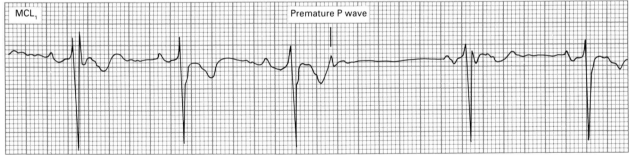

Sinus bradycardia with a blocked (nonconducted) premature atrial complex.

The blocked PAC is characterized by a regular rhythm interrupted by a pause, with a premature P wave occurring on or near the T wave of the preceding sequence. The premature P wave, which usually distorts the ST segment or T wave immediately before the pause, distinguishes this rhythm from a sinus arrest. PACs may be caused by hypoxemia, increased atrial pressure, or stimulant use. Initial treatment may consist of supplemental oxygen, identification and correction of the underlying cause, or antiarrhythmic drugs. Some PACs do not require treatment.

Atrial tachycardia

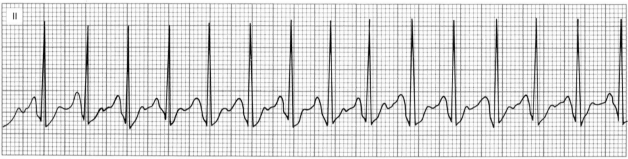

Atrial tachycardia with absolutely regular P-P intervals. Here, the heart rate is 160 beats/minute.

Atrial tachycardia occurs when an ectopic site in the atria takes over as pacemaker at an accelerated rate or a premature impulse from the atria sets off a reentry circuit within the atria. Atrial tachycardia is characterized by a normal P-QRS-T sequence with a rate between 150 and 250 beats/minute and absolutely regular P-P intervals. The absolute regularity and abnormal configuration of the P waves help differentiate this rhythm from sinus tachycardia. Using calipers, you can track the interval from one P wave to the next across the rhythm, even if some P waves become blocked in the conduction system.

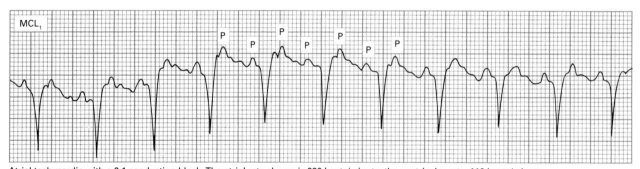

Atrial tachycardia with a 2:1 conduction block. The atrial rate shown is 220 beats/minute; the ventricular rate, 110 beats/minute.

An ECG strip usually will not show whether the reentry cycle is within the atria or from the atria to the ventricle or AV junction and back to the atria. Atrial tachycardia may be triggered by drug toxicity or by the same factors that cause PACs. Digoxin toxicity may cause an atrial tachycardia with a block or varying conduction. The characteristic rapid, regular P waves occur, but more than one P wave may be associated with each QRS complex.

Classified as a type of supraventricular tachycardia, atrial tachycardia commonly occurs as a paroxysmal rhythm with an abrupt onset or ending. Because of its rapid rate, the rhythm usually reduces cardiac output and may cause pallor, hypotension, dizziness, chest pain, palpitations, or syncope. Treatment may include vagal stimulation, oxygen, calcium channel blockers or beta blockers, or cardioversion. If associated with pump failure, the rhythm may be treated with digoxin, provided that digoxin toxicity is not the cause.

Atrial flutter and atrial fibrillation

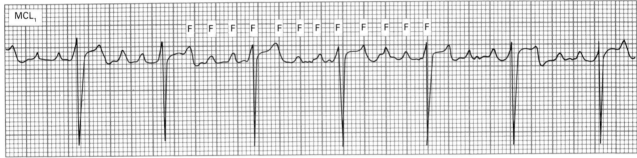

Atrial flutter with 4:1 conduction.

Atrial flutter is characterized by unusually shaped atrial depolarizations. The flutter waves (F waves) appear as "saw-tooth" or "picket-fence" P waves that occur 250 to 360 times per minute (most commonly, 300 beats/minute) at absolutely regular intervals. The atrial rate is faster than the ventricular rate, with the flutter waves occurring concurrently with the QRS complexes and T waves. This overlap may distort the QRS complex or the T wave. The wave sequence consists of an equal or unequal number of F waves occurring between QRS-T wave series and appears as F-F-FQRSFT-F-FQRSFT-F. One or more F waves may be hidden within the QRS complex or the T wave. If the conduction ratio of F waves to QRS complexes does not vary, the ventricular rate is regular. If the ratio varies, the ventricular rate is irregular. Common ratios of F waves to QRS complexes are 2:1, 3:1, and 4:1.

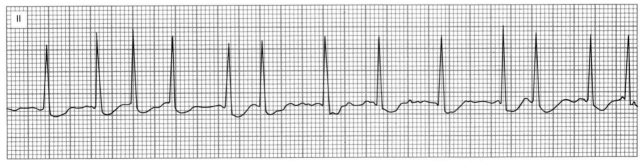

Atrial fibrillation with rapid or uncontrolled ventricular response. The rate shown is approximately 130 beats/minute.

In atrial fibrillation, multiple chaotic depolarizations occur in different atrial sites, producing a rapid, irregular series of atrial impulses. The atrial rate is indeterminate, with varying numbers of fibrillatory waves (f waves) occurring between each QRS-T sequence. These waves continue through ventricular depolarization and may distort the QRS complexes or T waves. Irregular conduction of the impulses to the ventricles results in a grossly irregular ventricular response and a wave sequence of fffQRSTfffffQRSTffQRSTf. Any number of f waves can occur between QRS complexes; the number does not stay constant.

Because the ventricular rate may vary dramatically from beat to beat, the best way to obtain an estimated rate from an ECG strip is to count the QRS complexes in a 6-second strip and multiply by 10; then repeat the process on one or more additional 6-second intervals and calculate an average rate. Ventricular rates over 100 beats/minute are said to be uncontrolled; those under 100 beats/minute usually reflect conduction that has been slowed or controlled by drug therapy. Slower rates allow more time for passive filling of the ventricle.

Atrial flutter and atrial fibrillation result in a loss of atrial contraction, or atrial kick, and usually decrease the patient's cardiac output. Both rhythms may be treated with antiarrhythmic drugs, digoxin (if the rhythm is associated with pump failure), or cardioversion.

Rhythms originating in the AV junction

Major rhythms associated with the AV junction include premature junctional complex, junctional rhythm, and supraventricular tachycardia.

Premature junctional complex

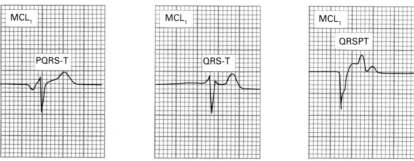

Patterns of premature junctional complex: PQRS-T, QRS-T, and QRSPT.

A premature junctional complex (PJC) is an early, ectopic impulse that arises in the AV junction. Like a PAC, for which it may be mistaken, a PJC appears as an early wave sequence disturbing the rhythm, but the position of the P wave differs. In a rhythm that originates in the AV junction, conduction to the atria (P wave) is caused by retrograde transmission of the current. This reverse AV node-to-atria conduction produces an inverted P wave in lead II and one of the following P wave patterns: a short P-R interval (PQRS-T) of less than 0.12 second if the P wave precedes the QRS complex, a P wave buried in the QRS complex (QRS-T), or a P wave after the QRS complex on the ST segment (QRSPT).

Junctional rhythm

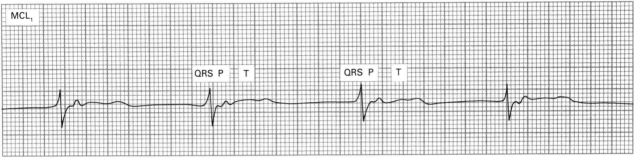

Junctional rhythm with an escape rate of approximately 42 beats/minute.

The AV junction can also serve as a backup pacemaker when the SA node fails to discharge, with an escape rate of 40 to 60 beats/minute. The slow rhythm, called junctional (or idiojunctional) rhythm, is treated with atropine if the patient develops symptoms, such as hypotension, ventricular ectopy, or altered mental status. If the AV junction becomes irritable, the rate may accelerate to 60 to 100 beats/minute. A junctional tachycardia would have the same wave sequence, but its rate would be between 100 and 180 beats/minute. Treatment for junctional tachycardia is the same as for atrial tachycardia.

Supraventricular tachycardia

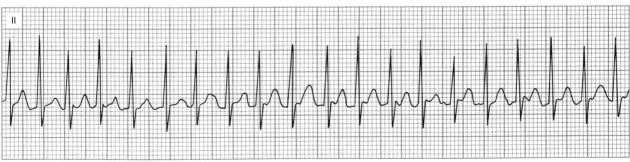

Supraventricular tachycardia with a rate of approximately 200 beats/minute.

Supraventricular tachycardia (SVT) is an absolutely regular ectopic tachycardia that originates above the ventricles and may include atrial tachycardia, junctional tachycardia, and atrial flutter with 1:1 or 2:1 conduction. If the rhythm begins and ends abruptly, it is called paroxysmal supraventricular tachycardia (PSVT). Symptoms of all the rhythms are similar. The fast rate generated by SVT usually decreases cardiac output by decreasing ventricular filling time. SVT also increases myocardial oxygen demand while coronary perfusion is diminishing. This may cause ischemia, precipitating angina pectoris. Other symptoms may include hypotension, palpitations, dizziness, or syncope.

Rhythms originating in the ventricles

Ventricular rhythms are characterized by widened, distorted QRS complexes (0.12 second or greater) and include premature ventricular complex, idioventricular rhythm, accelerated ventricular rhythm, ventricular tachycardia, and ventricular fibrillation.

Premature ventricular complex

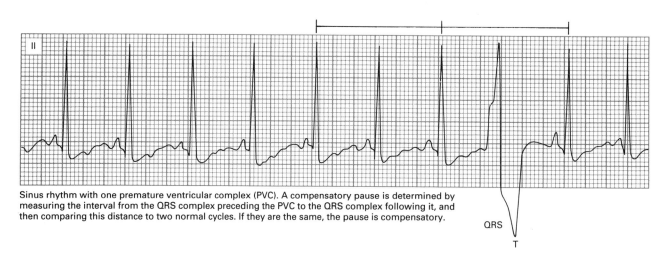

Sinus rhythm with one premature ventricular complex (PVC). A compensatory pause is determined by measuring the interval from the QRS complex preceding the PVC to the QRS complex following it, and then comparing this distance to two normal cycles. If they are the same, the pause is compensatory.

A premature ventricular complex (PVC), or premature ventricular depolarization, occurs early in the cycle and typically has a Q-R-S-T wave sequence. Usually, the T wave vector is opposite that of the QRS complex, and the premature series is followed by a compensatory pause. When a patient has more than one PVC, configurations of the QRS complexes are compared. If the configurations are the same, the PVCs are called unifocal or monomorphic:

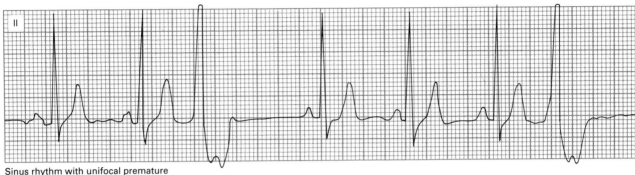

Sinus rhythm with unifocal premature ventricular complexes.

If the configurations differ, the PVCs are called multifocal or polymorphic:

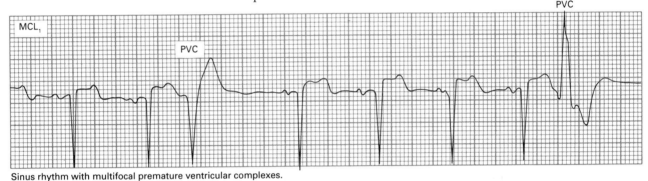

Sinus rhythm with multifocal premature ventricular complexes.

PVCs may occur in a particular pattern. If every other impulse is ectopic, the rhythm is called bigeminy; if every third impulse is ectopic, the rhythm is called trigeminy.

PVCs usually indicate ventricular irritability and can be a warning sign of life-threatening arrhythmias. Lidocaine (Xylocaine) is typically administered to treat PVCs when the patient has an acute cardiac condition, such as myocardial infarction. Other antiarrhythmic drugs that may be used include procainamide (Promine), quinidine (Duraquin), tocainide (Tonocard), and mexiletine (Mexitil).

Idioventricular rhythm

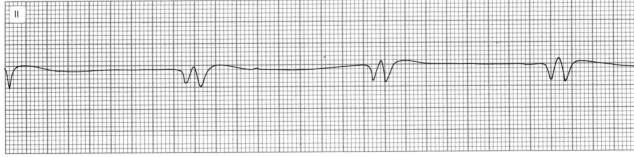

Idioventricular rhythm with a rate of about 32 beats/minute.

The ventricles act as a final backup pacemaker when both the SA node and the AV junction fail to initiate an impulse. An idioventricular rhythm is a slow, essentially regular rhythm that becomes slower and more irregular with time. The rate is usually in the range of 15 to 40 beats/minute, with a wave sequence of Q-R-S-T. The slow rate, the widened and distorted QRS complex, and the vector of the T wave distinguish this rhythm from junctional rhythm. As the rate becomes progressively slower, cardiac output diminishes dramatically; epinephrine, atropine, or pacing is required to sustain the patient's life.

Accelerated ventricular rhythm and ventricular tachycardia

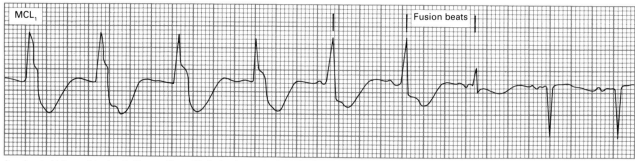

Accelerated idioventricular rhythm ending with fusion beats to sinus rhythm.

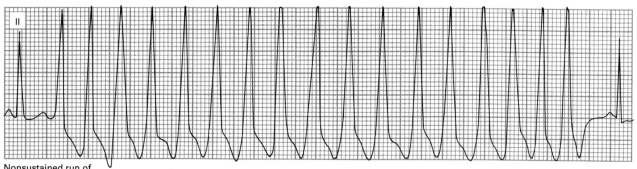

Nonsustained run of ventricular tachycardia.

Ectopic sites in the ventricle may become irritable and have increased automaticity, producing either an accelerated ventricular rhythm or ventricular tachycardia. Both are essentially regular rhythms with widened, distorted QRS complexes and T waves with opposite polarity. Occasionally, P waves appear, but these are unrelated to the QRS complexes, which are commonly monophasic or biphasic. If MCL_1 is used for monitoring, the QRS complex of a ventricular impulse would not be expected to be triphasic (RSR'). The wave sequence for ventricular tachycardia might be Q-S-T-Q-S-T or R-S-T-R-S-T.

Accelerated ventricular rhythm has a ventricular rate of 40 to 100 beats/minute and commonly maintains adequate cardiac output. In contrast, ventricular tachycardia is characterized by a ventricular rate of 100 to 200 beats/minute, usually adversely affecting cardiac output. The rhythm may or may not produce cardiac output and pulses in the patient, stressing the importance of careful patient assessment. Treatment usually consists of antiarrhythmic drug therapy for a stable patient and cardioversion for an unstable patient. If the patient has no pulse, either cardiopulmonary resuscitation (CPR) or defibrillation is necessary.

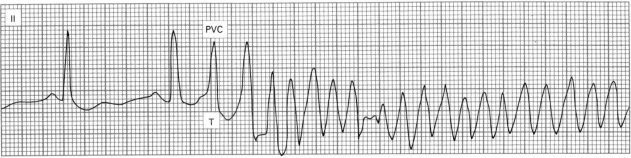

Sinus bradycardia followed by an R-on-T phenomenon that initiates torsades de pointes.

Torsades de pointes, an atypical form of ventricular tachycardia, has a regular rate above 200 beats/minute and QRS complexes that appear to twist around the baseline. This twisting effect causes the height of the QRS complexes to decrease and increase gradually as the rhythm progresses. Torsades de pointes is usually initiated by an R-on-T phenomenon, in which the R wave of a PVC occurs on the vulnerable phase of a T wave preceding it. The rhythm is sometimes associated with Class 1A antiarrhythmic drug toxicity, hypokalemia, hypomagnesemia, and psychotropic drugs (phenothiazines and tricyclic antidepressants), which lengthen the QT interval. Commonly, the rhythm is nonsustained, and the patient spontaneously converts to his normal rhythm. A sustained rhythm may progress to ventricular fibrillation. Treatment may consist of antiarrhythmic drugs, pacing, defibrillation, isoproterenol (Isuprel), or correction of underlying electrolyte imbalances.

Ventricular fibrillation

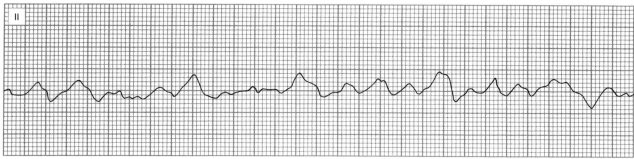

Ventricular fibrillation.

Ventricular fibrillation (VF) is a chaotic rhythm without recognizable QRS complexes or T waves. In their place appear grossly irregular undulations of the baseline, representing disorganized depolarizations of small areas within the ventricles. No single impulse is strong enough to depolarize a critical mass of myocardium. Because VF is ineffective in producing cardiac output or pulses, the rhythm is life-threatening and demands immediate recognition and treatment with CPR and defibrillation.

Asystole

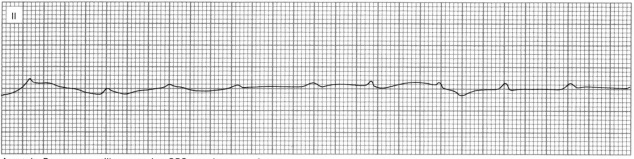

Asystole. P waves are still present, but QRS complexes are absent.

Asystole is the absence of organized electrical activity in the heart, represented on an ECG recording as a flattened, almost straight baseline. Because a completely straight line usually signals a mechanical problem, such as a loose electrode, always assess the patient for absent pulses before assuming asystole. A slightly wavy baseline may mask fine VF, so check a second monitoring lead to verify asystole.

Atrioventricular blocks

The AV junction is the only normal conduction pathway from the atria to the ventricular conduction system. A delay or blockage of transmission of impulses to the ventricles results in a first-, second-, or third-degree AV block, categorized according to severity.

First-degree AV block

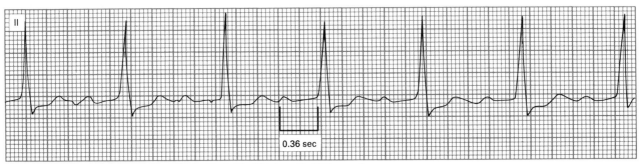

Sinus rhythm with first-degree atrioventricular block. The PR interval is 0.36 second.

A first-degree AV block may occur with any sinus mechanism and is manifested by a PR interval greater than 0.20 second. A prolonged return to the isoelectric baseline after the P wave creates a P—QRS-T wave sequence.

Second-degree AV block

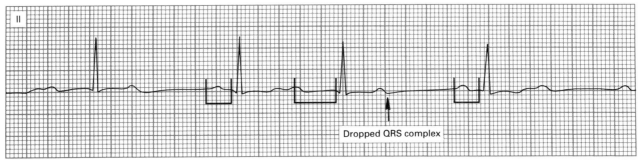

Second-degree atrioventricular block Type I. The PR interval progresses from 0.26 second to 0.47 second, and then the P wave is blocked. The next PR interval is 0.26 second.

A second-degree AV block indicates a greater degree of impulse blocking so that not all P waves are conducted to the ventricles. Type I, also called Wenckebach or Mobitz I, is characterized by a regular atrial rhythm (P-P interval) and an irregular ventricular rhythm. P waves outnumber QRS complexes, and the rhythm seems to have a patterned regularity. The PR interval gradually lengthens as the R-R intervals shorten until, finally, one P wave is not followed by a QRS complex. The next P wave is conducted with a PR interval that is shorter than the one preceding the nonconducted P wave. This cycle tends to repeat itself, with each group of beats having one more P wave than QRS complex. Thus, the wave sequence is P-QRS-T-P—QRS-TP———P-QRS-T. This rhythm is usually transient, and the patient may not need treatment.

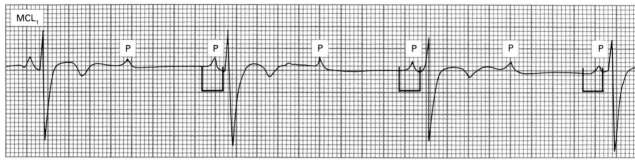

Second-degree atrioventricular block Type II with a consistent PR interval of 0.15 second.

Type II, also called Mobitz II, usually indicates a pathologic condition or blockage in the bundle of His and is commonly associated with a bundle branch block. Characteristics of Type II include a regular atrial rhythm, more P waves than QRS complexes, and PR intervals that remain consistent whenever P waves are conducted (although any number of P waves may be nonconducted). This rhythm may produce a regular ventricular rate if the conduction ratio of P waves to QRS complexes remains constant or an irregular rate if the ratio varies. The wave sequence would appear as P———P-QRS-TP———P-QRS-TP. Type II usually causes a significant drop in heart rate and cardiac output.

Both types of second-degree block may be caused by ischemia or drug toxicity. Drug therapy or pacing is indicated if the patient develops symptoms, such as hypotension, syncope, or ventricular ectopy.

Third-degree AV block

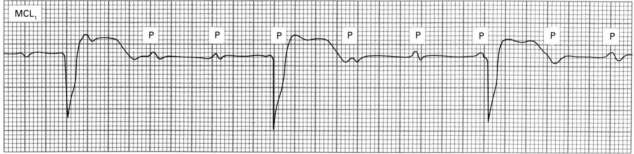

Third-degree atrioventricular block. The atrial rate shown is 95 beats/minute; the ventricular rate, 30 beats/minute.

A third-degree AV block, or complete heart block, is a cessation of conduction from the atria to the ventricles and usually constitutes an emergency. The rhythm is easily recognized by the complete absence of a relationship between the P waves and the QRS complexes. AV dissociation is produced. In third-degree AV block, the ventricular rate is slower than the atrial rate, and P waves may be superimposed on the QRS complexes and T waves, typically distorting these waves.

Essentially, the atria and the ventricles act as two separate conduction systems, each with its own pacemaker. The ventricular pacemaker may be the AV junction or a site within the ventricles. A rhythm from the junction usually has a rate of 40 to 60 beats/minute and a normal QRS complex duration. A rhythm produced by a site in the ventricles usually has a rate of less than 40 beats/minute and QRS complex durations greater than 0.12 second. The atrial pacemaker may be the sinus node or an ectopic atrial focus. The usual pattern is P——P—QRPS-T-P——PQRS-TP.

Correlating the rhythm to the patient's condition

Besides correctly identifying the ECG rhythm, you must accurately assess the patient. Physical findings should be appropriate for the rhythm interpretation. For example, neither asystole nor VF would be an appropriate rhythm interpretation for a patient who is alert and awake, with a pulse of 80 beats/minute and a blood pressure of 100/60 mm Hg. In this instance, check the monitoring system to ensure that electrodes were correctly applied and that the system is operating properly.

Occasionally, a rhythm on the monitor indicates that the patient should have a pulse even though careful assessment reveals that the patient is pulseless. This condition, referred to as electromechanical dissociation (EMD), demands that the underlying cause of the lack of cardiac output be determined and corrected. EMD is classified as primary or secondary and may be associated with severe myocardial depression late in a code or may be caused by hypovolemia, tension pneumothorax, or cardiac tamponade, all of which decrease ventricular filling. CPR should be performed until the problem is corrected. (See Chapter 10, Electromechanical Dissociation, for a more detailed discussion.)

5

Pharmacologic Therapy

Pharmacologic intervention is an integral part of cardiac emergency treatment. Drugs may be administered to correct hypoxemia, reestablish spontaneous circulation, optimize cardiac function, suppress sustained ventricular arrhythmia, correct acidosis, relieve pain, or treat congestive heart failure (CHF). This chapter presents the pharmacology of drugs commonly used during cardiac emergencies, including inotropic and vasoactive drugs, antiarrhythmics, and miscellaneous drugs.

Inotropic and vasoactive drugs

Some drugs, such as the antiarrhythmic propranolol, have a negative inotropic effect; that is, they decrease myocardial contractility. Other drugs, such as the adrenergic receptor dobutamine, have a positive inotropic effect; that is, they increase myocardial contractility. Inotropic drugs, then, directly or indirectly augment cardiac output. Vasoactive drugs dilate or constrict the blood vessels. Many of these drugs, called *sympathomimetic* because their actions mimic the action of the sympathetic nervous system, exert their action at the system's neuroeffector junction.

Adrenergic receptors

Sympathetic nervous system receptors are called *adrenergic* because nerve impulses are usually transmitted to the effector cells by the release of no r*adren*alin (norepinephrine). The three types of adrenergic receptors — alpha-adrenergic, beta-adrenergic, and dopaminergic — are affected by different drugs used in cardiac emergencies.

Alpha-adrenergic receptors are present mainly in neurons located in vascular smooth muscle. Stimulation of these receptors leads to vasoconstriction. Alpha$_2$ receptors, which can be considered "modulators," provide a countereffect for the alpha$_1$ receptors. When the alpha$_2$ receptors are stimulated, norepinephrine release at the nerve endings decreases, leading to blood vessel dilation.

Beta$_1$ receptors are located primarily in the myocardial muscle and the cardiac conduction system. Their stimulation increases myocardial contractility and the heart rate. Beta$_2$ receptors of importance in cardiac emergencies are located in blood vessels and bronchial smooth muscle. Their stimulation leads to vasodilation and relaxation of bronchial smooth muscle and also causes glycogenolysis (breakdown of glycogen stores in the liver) and intracellular potassium movement.

Dopaminergic receptors are located in renal, mesenteric, coronary, and intracerebral vascular beds. Stimulation of these receptors causes vasodilation and increased blood flow.

Cardiac output determinants

Cardiac output is a product of the heart rate and the stroke volume. Alteration of either affects cardiac output, which is the objective of the inotropic and vasoactive drugs. The three main factors that determine stroke volume are preload, afterload, and contractility. *Preload* is the ventricular volume and pressure at the end of diastole. Either excessive or inadequate preload adversely affects cardiac output and increases oxygen demand. *Afterload* is the resistance against which the heart has to pump. It reflects systemic vascular resistance (SVR) or the amount of resistance (vasoconstriction) in the

SELECTED DRUGS USED IN CARDIAC EMERGENCIES

INOTROPIC AND VASOACTIVE DRUGS

Adrenergic receptor stimulators
epinephrine (Adrenalin)
norepinephrine (Levophed)
dopamine hydrochloride (Intropin)
dobutamine (Dobutrex)
isoproterenol (Isuprel)

Cardiac glycoside
digoxin (Lanoxin)

Vasodilators
nitroprusside sodium (Nipride)
nitroglycerin (Nitrostat)

Other
amrinone (Inocor)

ANTIARRHYTHMIC DRUGS

Class I
Group A
quinidine (Quinidex)
procainamide (Pronestyl)
disopyramide (Norpace)

Group B
lidocaine (Xylocaine)
tocainide (Tonocard)
phenytoin (Dilantin)

Group C
flecainide (Tambocor)

Class II
propranolol (Inderal)
metoprolol (Lopressor)
atenolol (Tenormin)
acebutolol (Sectral)
timolol (Blocadren)

Class III
bretylium (Bretylol)
amiodarone (Cordarone)

Class IV
verapamil (Calan)
diltiazem (Cardizem)

MISCELLANEOUS DRUGS

atropine
sodium bicarbonate
morphine sulfate
calcium chloride
oxygen

peripheral blood vessels. Increases in afterload not only increase oxygen demand (the heart has to use more energy to eject the blood) but also indirectly decrease cardiac output if the heart cannot maintain increased contractile strength to eject the blood against increased resistance. *Contractility* refers to the ventricles' ability to contract. Increased contractility increases cardiac output but also increases myocardial oxygen consumption.

Maintaining a balance between myocardial oxygen supply and demand is critical to the patient's health. Many inotropic drugs increase cardiac output but at the same time increase myocardial oxygen demand and consumption. Optimizing heart rate, preload, afterload, and contractility is the key to optimizing cardiac performance.

HEMODYNAMIC EFFECTS OF SELECTED INOTROPIC AND VASOACTIVE DRUGS

Drug	Heart Rate	Preload	Afterload	Contractility
epinephrine (Adrenalin)	Increases	Increases	May increase or decrease	Increases
norepinephrine (Levophed)	May increase or decrease	Increases	Increases	Increases
dopamine (Intropin)	May increase or decrease	Decreases	May increase	Increases
dobutamine (Dobutrex)	May increase	Decreases	May increase or decrease	Increases
isoproterenol (Isuprel)	Increases	Decreases	Decreases	Increases
digoxin (Lanoxin)	May decrease	Has no effect	May increase or decrease	Increases
amrinone (Inocor)	May increase	Decreases	Decreases	Increases
nitroprusside (Nipride)	May increase	Decreases	Decreases	Has no effect
nitroglycerin (Nitrostat)	May increase	Decreases	Decreases	Has no effect

Epinephrine

Epinephrine is an endogenous catecholamine (a hormone produced by the body) that stimulates both alpha- and beta-adrenergic receptors. Physiologic stimuli, such as stress and exercise, increase endogenous secretion. The effects of epinephrine (Adrenalin) administration can vary, depending on the body's response to the drug. For instance, if cardiac output decreases, the body's reflex response is to secrete epinephrine, which stimulates beta$_1$ receptors. Common effects of epinephrine, whether endogenous or exogenously administered, include elevated arterial blood pressure and increased systemic resistance, heart rate, myocardial contractility, automaticity, and coronary and cerebral blood flow—all of which subsequently raise myocardial oxygen consumption. Additionally, epinephrine may make the ventricular myocardium more receptive to defibrillation by increasing the amplitude of ventricular fibrillation, although this effect is not widely documented (Otto, 1986).

Indications
Ventricular fibrillation (especially effective with fine VF), asystole, electromechanical dissociation.

Dosages
0.5 to 1 mg (5 to 10 ml of a 1:10,000 solution) every 5 minutes I.V. or 1 mg every 5 minutes by the endotracheal route. Optimal dose in cardiac arrest may be 3 to 5 mg (Gonzalez et al., 1989).

Precautions
• Can provoke arrhythmias, such as tachycardias and ventricular ectopy.
• Increases myocardial oxygen demand, which may precipitate myocardial ischemia.

Norepinephrine
Norepinephrine (Levophed) is an endogenous catecholamine with predominantly alpha-adrenergic effects. It is a potent alpha-receptor stimulator, producing arterial and venous vasoconstriction, and exerts minimal beta$_2$ effects. Additionally, norepinephrine exerts a positive inotropic effect through beta$_1$ stimulation, thus increasing myocardial contractility.

Indications
Hemodynamically significant hypotension or cardiogenic shock. Particularly helpful with low SVR.

Dosages
Initially, 8 mcg/minute; titrate for desired result. Usual adult dose is 2 to 12 mcg/minute, although higher doses may be needed.

Precautions
• Contraindicated in hypovolemia.
• Increases myocardial oxygen demand without increasing coronary artery blood flow.
• Causes renal and mesenteric vasoconstriction.
• Also causes tissue necrosis and subsequent sloughing if extravasation occurs; low concentrations of an alpha antagonist, such as phentolamine (Regitine), may be added to the I.V. infusion of norepinephrine to prevent tissue necrosis.

Dopamine hydrochloride
Dopamine (Intropin), a chemical precursor of norepinephrine, stimulates beta$_1$, alpha, and dopaminergic receptors. Its effects are dose-dependent. In low doses (1 to 2 mcg/kg/minute), dopamine stimulates vascular D$_1$ dopaminergic receptors, causing renal, mesenteric, and coronary artery dilation that increases urine output, the desired effect. At doses of 2 to 10 mcg/kg/minute, dopamine stimu-

lates beta$_1$ receptors, increasing myocardial contractility and thus cardiac output. At higher doses (10 to 20 mcg/kg/minute), the alpha$_1$ effects predominate, increasing SVR and preload by peripheral arterial and venous vasoconstriction. At doses above 20 mcg/kg/minute, dopamine has effects similar to those of norepinephrine.

Indications
Cardiogenic shock, hemodynamically significant hypotension.

Dosages
2 to 5 mcg/kg/minute; titrate for desired effect. Use the lowest dose necessary to achieve desired results.

Precautions
• Contraindicated in hypovolemia.
• May induce arrhythmias.
• With higher doses, may precipitate ischemia and chest pain.
• Nausea and vomiting are common.
• Do not add to alkaline I.V. solutions.
• May cause tissue damage if infiltration occurs.
• Administer dopamine through a central I.V. line rather than a peripheral one.

Dobutamine hydrochloride
Dobutamine (Dobutrex), a synthetic catecholamine, stimulates beta$_1$ adrenergic receptors, exerting no significant effects on beta$_2$ or alpha receptors. The drug acts directly on the heart muscle to increase the strength of myocardial contraction; it only minimally affects heart rate and blood pressure. Peripheral resistance and heart rate usually fall reflexively because of an increase in cardiac output (increased cardiac output reflexively decreases catecholamine release, which causes vasoconstriction and increased heart rate). Because dobutamine increases myocardial contractility without increasing peripheral resistance, it increases oxygen demand to a lesser degree than other drugs.

Indications
Refractory heart failure, pulmonary congestion.

Dosages
Initially, 0.5 mcg/kg/minute by I.V. drip; titrate for desired effect. Usual dose is 2.5 to 20 mcg/kg/minute.

Precautions
May induce tachycardia, myocardial ischemia, headache, and nausea.

Isoproterenol hydrochloride

Isoproterenol (Isuprel) is a synthetic sympathomimetic drug with potent nonselective beta-agonist properties. It has little effect on beta receptors. The drug increases both the rate and strength of myocardial contraction, which commonly increases cardiac output and decreases SVR from beta$_2$ vasodilation and venous pooling. However, because isoproterenol greatly increases myocardial oxygen demand and may induce myocardial ischemia, its use is limited.

Indications

Hemodynamically significant, atropine-refractory bradycardia.

Dosages

2 to 10 mcg/minute; titrate for desired effect.

Precautions

• Contraindicated in cardiac arrest.
• May increase myocardial oxygen consumption.
• May induce severe arrhythmias.

Amrinone lactate

Amrinone (Inocor), an inotropic agent that also has vasodilator effects, inhibits the breakdown of cyclic adenosine monophosphate (AMP) into its inactive form. Cyclic AMP promotes calcium entry into muscle cells and thus increases contractile strength. Because the drug does not directly stimulate adrenergic receptors, its effects cannot be reversed by adrenergic-blocking drugs. Amrinone's hemodynamic effects are similar to those of dobutamine: cardiac output increases, and SVR and preload diminish.

Indications

CHF refractory to conventional inotropic agents.

Dosages

Loading dose 0.75 mg/kg over 2 to 3 minutes; follow with I.V. infusion of 5 to 10 mcg/kg/minute.

Precautions

Can worsen myocardial ischemia. Use lowest possible dose.

Digoxin

Digoxin (Lanoxin) exerts a positive inotropic effect by inhibiting sodium-potassium ATPase, the "sodium pump." Intracellular sodium rises slightly, activating a mechanism that exchanges extracellular calcium for intracellular sodium. The net effect is an increase in calcium available for muscle contraction. This effect is not inhibited by adrenergic blockers (such as propranolol) because the drug does not directly stimulate adrenergic receptors. Additionally, digoxin suppresses sinoatrial (SA) node automaticity and depresses impulse conduction through the atrioventricular (AV) node.

Indications
May be useful in treating CHF and refractory paroxysmal supraventricular tachycardia. Has limited use in emergency cardiac care setting.

Dosages
Dose depends on administration route and desired effect. Loading dose is usually 10 to 15 mcg/kg (0.5 to 1 mg); maintenance dose is usually 0.125 to 0.5 mg daily.

Precautions
• Toxicity is common.
• Guard against hypokalemia, which precipitates digoxin toxicity.
• Can cause GI irritation and central nervous system (CNS) disturbances.

Nitroprusside sodium
Nitroprusside (Nipride), a potent peripheral vasodilator, affects both arterial and venous circulation. The drug has a rapid onset, and its action ceases within minutes of stopping the infusion. Nitroprusside decreases SVR (afterload)—thus indirectly increasing cardiac output—and increases venous capacitance (preload).

Indications
Cardiogenic pulmonary edema, hypertensive crisis.

Dosages
0.5 to 8 mcg/kg/minute; titrate for desired effect.

Precautions
• Can cause sudden and profound hypotension.
• Can lead to cyanide toxicity (the drug is metabolized by red blood cells to hydrocyanic acid, which the liver converts to thiocyanate).

Nitroglycerin
Nitroglycerin (Nitrostat, Tridil) is a vascular smooth-muscle relaxant that dilates large coronary arteries, antagonizes vasospasm, and stimulates coronary collateral blood flow to the myocardium. It also causes peripheral vasodilation, thus lowering preload and afterload.

Indications
Commonly used for angina. May have benefit in acute myocardial infarction (MI) and CHF.

Dosages

0.3 to 0.6 mg by sublingual tablet every 3 to 5 minutes (maximum of three doses) or 10 to 20 mcg/minute by I.V. drip, titrated for effect.

Precautions

May cause hypotension (secondary to vasodilation), headache, bradycardia, methemoglobinemia (as the drug is metabolized).

Antiarrhythmic drugs

Antiarrhythmic drug therapy is initiated to restore normal cardiac rhythm and to prevent recurrence of an arrhythmia. Antiarrhythmic drugs vary in action and effect on various arrhythmias and are commonly divided into four classes, according to their mechanism of action. Class I antiarrhythmics are membrane-depressant drugs that slow sodium influx during depolarization. Class II antiarrhythmics are beta-adrenergic blockers that compete with beta-adrenergic stimulators at receptor sites. Class III antiarrhythmics prolong repolarization, thus decreasing the potential for premature impulse formation. Class IV antiarrhythmics are calcium channel blockers.

Lidocaine hydrochloride

Lidocaine (Xylocaine), a class IB agent, is used for managing ventricular ectopy. It decreases excessive automaticity of ectopic pacemakers by slowing the rate of depolarization. Specifically, lidocaine slows the entry of sodium through the fast channels, decreases excitability, and lengthens the effective refractory period. It has little if any effect on conduction velocity.

Indications

Premature ventricular complex, ventricular tachycardia (VT), VF, prophylaxis in patients suspected of having an MI or ischemia, which reduces the fibrillation threshold.

Dosages

1 mg/kg by I.V. bolus or through endotracheal tube. Usual dose is 50 to 100 mg by I.V. bolus. Administer 0.5 mg/kg boluses every 5 to 10 minutes, as necessary, up to 3 mg/kg. Follow suppression of arrhythmia with a continuous I.V. drip of 2 to 4 mg/minute.

Precautions

• Reduced dose may be needed in elderly patients and in those with heart failure or shock.
• CNS toxic reactions are not uncommon.
• Use with caution in patients with conduction disturbances.
• Toxic effects are mainly seen as CNS disturbances.

Procainamide hydrochloride

Procainamide (Pronestyl) is a class IA drug that suppresses ventricular ectopic impulses. It decreases the slope of phase 4 diastolic depolarization, which reduces the automaticity of ectopic pacemakers in the ventricular muscle and Purkinje fibers. Procainamide also slows conduction by decreasing the slope of phase 0 of the action potential.

Indications

Suppression of ventricular ectopy unresponsive to lidocaine.

Dosages

20 mg I.V. every minute or 100 mg every 5 minutes up to the maximum dose of 1,000 mg. Follow suppression with a continuous I.V. drip of 2 to 4 mg/minute. Discontinue the I.V. bolus if the QRS complex widens more than 50%, the patient's blood pressure decreases, the total dose of 1 g is administered, or ectopy is suppressed.

Precautions

QRS widening and precipitous hypotension can occur.

Quinidine sulfate

Quinidine (Quinidex) is a Class IA antiarrhythmic. Like other Class I drugs, it slows the flow of sodium into the cell, lengthens the refractory period, and slows conduction velocity. Quinidine decreases contractile strength, however, and can cause vasodilation.

Indications

Especially effective for atrial fibrillation and atrial flutter. Also used for most supraventricular arrhythmias not associated with heart block.

Dosages

200 to 300 mg orally 3 to 4 times daily. Maximum daily dose should not exceed 4 g. Depending on serum drug levels, dosage may need to be decreased for patients with CHF, a hepatic disorder, or renal failure.

Precautions

• May increase digoxin toxicity.
• Because the drug decreases contractility, use is limited in patients with heart failure.
• GI irritation may be a sign of quinidine toxicity.
• Contraindicated in patients with AV blocks or conduction defects.
• Allergic reactions are not uncommon.

Propranolol

Propranolol (Inderal), a Class II antiarrhythmic, blocks the action of catecholamines at beta $_1$ and beta $_2$ receptors. The drug may help control arrhythmias that are in part caused by catecholamine stimulation. Propranolol also reduces AV nodal conduction and therefore slows ventricular responses to arrhythmias, such as atrial fibrillation and atrial flutter.

Indications

Recurrent VT or VF, paroxysmal supraventricular tachycardia.

Dosages

For emergencies, 1 to 3 mg by slow I.V. drip while monitoring the patient's blood pressure. Oral dose is 10 to 30 mg three to four times daily.

Precautions
• May cause or worsen heart failure, bronchospasm, and hypotension.
• May produce or increase AV block.
• May cause GI irritation or CNS disturbances.

Bretylium tosylate

Bretylium (Bretylol) is a Class III drug that lengthens the duration of the action potential. This increases the refractory period and decreases the chance of premature impulses. Bretylium also increases the threshold for VF and blocks post-ganglionic nerve endings, which produces hypotension.

Indications

VT and VF resistant to lidocaine and defibrillation, recurrent VF after lidocaine therapy, failure to control unstable VT.

Dosages

5 mg/kg by I.V. bolus followed by 10 mg/kg every 10 to 15 minutes up to 30 mg/kg. Average dose is 350 mg by I.V. bolus.

Precautions
• Can cause postural hypotension.
• Commonly causes nausea and vomiting in conscious patients.
• Can aggravate digoxin toxicity.

Verapamil

Verapamil (Calan) is a Class IV antiarrhythmic that suppresses the slow calcium channels. It slows conduction velocity, prolongs the refractory period of the AV node, and induces coronary artery vasodilation.

Indications
Paroxysmal supraventricular tachycardia.

Dosages
Initially, 5 mg I.V. If no response after 10 to 30 minutes, administer 10 mg.

Precautions
- May cause bradycardia and hypotension.
- May worsen or cause CHF.
- Contraindicated in most forms of VT.

Miscellaneous drugs
Miscellaneous drugs used to manage cardiac emergencies include atropine sulfate, sodium bicarbonate, morphine sulfate, calcium chloride, and oxygen.

Atropine sulfate
This parasympatholytic (sometimes called vagolytic) agent is commonly used in cardiac emergencies. By blocking parasympathetic receptors in the heart, atropine increases the SA node discharge rate and improves the AV node conduction rate, thus increasing the heart rate (see Chapter 1, The Heart: Anatomy and Physiology, for a review of parasympathetic nervous system actions). Atropine is used in symptomatic bradycardia and second- and third-degree heart blocks. The drug is sometimes administered to patients with asystole, although its beneficial effects are uncertain.

Indications
Hemodynamically significant bradycardia, asystole, pulseless idioventricular rhythms. May help decrease AV block.

Dosages
0.5 mg every 5 minutes. Complete vagolytic dose is 2 mg. Initial dose in asystole is 1 mg.

Precautions
- May worsen cardiac ischemia.
- May cause VF or VT.
- Do *not* use for asymptomatic bradycardia. Small doses (less than 0.5 mg) may paradoxically slow heart rate.

Sodium bicarbonate
This drug is administered to correct metabolic acidosis, which can develop during a cardiac arrest if chest compressions and artificial ventilations fail to maintain adequate circulation and oxygenation.

Administration in cardiac arrest is not recommended unless the acidosis is life-threatening and other modalities fail to correct it.

Indications
Severe metabolic acidosis that persists despite adequate chest compressions and artificial ventilations.

Dosages
1 mEq/kg by I.V. push, then 0.5 mEq every 10 minutes, depending on arterial blood gas values. Usual initial dose is 50 to 100 mEq.

Precautions
• Causes shifts in O_2 dissociation curve and increases hemoglobin affinity for oxygen.
• Induces hyperosmolarity, hypernatremia, paradoxical intracellular acidosis, and extracellular alkalosis.

Morphine sulfate
A potent narcotic analgesic, morphine sulfate is used primarily to control pain and, in cardiac emergencies, to increase venous capacitance and lower SVR.

Indications
Pain accompanying acute MI, acute pulmonary edema.

Dosages
2 to 5 mg I.V. every 5 minutes, titrated for effect.

Precautions
May cause respiratory depression and hypotension.

Oxygen
Oxygen administration plays a vital role in life support by relieving hypoxemia and increasing oxygen availability to the myocardium during cardiac emergencies.

Indications
Acute chest pain, suspected hypoxemia, cardiopulmonary arrest.

Dosages
As patient's condition warrants (for instance, 100% during a cardiopulmonary arrest).

Precautions
• Guided by arterial blood gas (ABG) values, decrease the amount of oxygen as soon as possible to prevent oxygen intoxication.
• Humidify oxygen as soon as possible to prevent tissue damage.
• Regularly assess ABG values to determine whether oxygen levels can be decreased.

6

Electrical and Mechanical Interventions

Although pharmacologic therapy can prevent or treat many cardiac problems, you must be prepared to use other emergency measures. This chapter reviews the electrical and mechanical interventions used to convert cardiac arrhythmias: cardiopulmonary resuscitation, defibrillation, cardioversion, precordial thump, and cardiac pacing.

Cardiopulmonary resuscitation

When breathing and circulation cease, cells throughout the body become oxygen-starved, unable to maintain normal metabolism. Excessive production of lactic and pyruvic acid leads to cellular necrosis. The success of advanced cardiac life support (ACLS) interventions depends on early recognition of this life-threatening situation. Cardiopulmonary resuscitation (CPR) helps maintain the circulation of oxygenated blood to tissues and organs, albeit at a rate about one-quarter to one-third of normal cardiac output. However, even this reduced cardiac output—if achieved quickly after a cardiac arrest—promotes the effectiveness of defibrillation, drug administration, and other therapeutic interventions.

Advanced adjunctive therapies, once available, should be employed along with CPR. For instance, as soon as supplemental oxygen is available, the patient should be ventilated with a manual bag-valve-mask system with 100% oxygen. Endotracheal intubation would be performed to protect and maintain an adequate airway if the patient remained unresponsive.

Cardiac compressions used during CPR generate cardiac output by changing intrathoracic pressures during compression and relaxation. This change in pressure creates gradients that permit blood flow. A similar change in intrathoracic pressure can be achieved by having a patient cough. For instance, frequent coughing has helped maintain consciousness in a patient experiencing an arrhythmia (which would normally cause loss of cardiac output) and has been demonstrated to convert ventricular tachycardia, complete heart block, and ventricular fibrillation. Coughing may one day be used more widely to convert abnormal rhythms.

Many abnormal rhythms require treatment other than with drugs. These treatments—defibrillation, cardioversion, precordial thump, and cardiac pacing—use electrical current to disrupt chaotic rhythms or stimulate cardiac electrical activity.

When chaotic activity, such as ventricular fibrillation, occurs, the sinus node cannot establish dominance as the normal pacemaker. The sinus impulse may still occur, but it becomes blocked in the fibrillating myocardium. For the sinus node to reestablish itself as the dominant pacemaker, the chaotic rhythm must be interrupted. This can be achieved by delivering an electrical current through the heart to depolarize all the cells simultaneously:

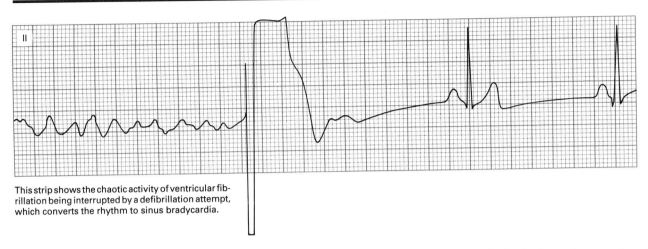

This strip shows the chaotic activity of ventricular fibrillation being interrupted by a defibrillation attempt, which converts the rhythm to sinus bradycardia.

As the cells repolarize (recover), the ones with the highest degree of automaticity should reach threshold first and discharge, thus establishing pacing dominance.

Defibrillation

The process of delivering an electrical current through the heart is called *defibrillation,* or *electrical countershock.* A defibrillator converts alternating current from an electrical outlet and delivers it to the patient as direct current through paddles applied to the chest. The amount of energy delivered (measured in joules, or watt-seconds) is sufficient to depolarize all cardiac cells within a few milliseconds. Portable defibrillators use a battery as the energy source.

The chest wall normally offers some resistance to the electrical current, but using conducting gel or defibrillator pads between the paddles and the chest decreases that resistance. A small amount of gel is applied to one paddle, and the paddles are rubbed together to coat both surfaces completely. Gel needs replacing after several defibrillations because it dries out. Another disadvantage is that, because it makes the chest slippery during chest compressions, the gel may need to be wiped off the chest between defibrillations. Defibrillator pads are easier to use because they adhere to the chest and usually last through multiple defibrillations.

Do not allow gel to create a "bridge" between the two paddles, because current will follow the path of least resistance and travel along the gel pathway rather than through the patient. Use firm pressure on the paddles. Each defibrillation lowers the resistance for any subsequent defibrillation. Therefore, during initial defibrillation, three successive countershocks are used before other interventions are attempted.

Paddle placement is also important. Most defibrillators permit direct monitoring through the paddles to obtain an immediate view of the electrocardiogram (ECG) rhythm on the monitor. These "quick-look" paddles are usually applied to the anterior chest in the defibrillation position: one paddle on the lower left chest at the cardiac apex and the other on the upper right chest near the sternum.

SCHEMATIC REPRESENTATION OF PADDLE PLACE-MENT FOR DEFIBRILLATION

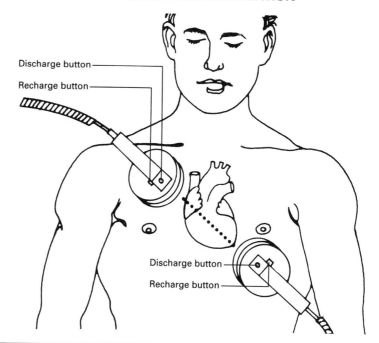

Discharge button

Recharge button

Discharge button

Recharge button

An alternate paddle placement (anterior-posterior) requiring different paddles is particularly effective for cardioversion. One paddle is placed over the heart on the anterior chest, and the other, a flat paddle, is placed under the patient's back beneath the left scapula.

PADDLE PLACEMENT FOR CARDIOVERSION

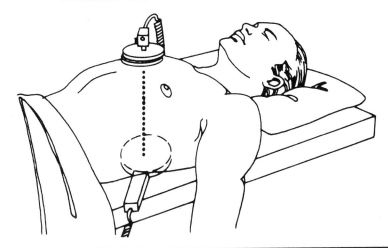

Although regular paddles may be used for anterior-posterior placement, the patient must be positioned on his side because the operator needs access to place the paddles and push the discharge buttons simultaneously. This placement is difficult to maintain unless the patient is an infant or small child.

The safety of the health care team during defibrillation must also be considered. Before discharging current from the paddles, the operator should ensure that no one is touching either the patient or anything in contact with him and then instruct everyone to "stand clear."

The initial energy level used to defibrillate an adult is 200 joules (or watt-seconds). If this is ineffective, the energy level is increased to 200 to 300 joules for the second defibrillation and to 360 joules for the third. In infants and children, the initial energy level is 2 joules/kg and may be doubled for repeat defibrillations.

PROCEDURE FOR DEFIBRILLATION
- Identify ventricular fibrillation or pulseless ventricular tachycardia on the monitor.
- Verify that the patient is pulseless.
- Apply defibrillation pads or gel.
- Charge the defibrillator to the desired energy level (initially, 200 joules for an adult).
- Place the paddles on the chest with firm pressure.
- Instruct the code team to "stand clear," and ensure that no one is in contact with the patient.
- Depress the buttons on both paddles simultaneously.
- Reassess the rhythm on the monitor.
- Check the patient's pulse.
- If defibrillation is unsuccessful, repeat the procedure.

Automatic defibrillators

Automatic defibrillators have proven effective in emergencies that occur outside the hospital. When applied to a pulseless person, the device automatically diagnoses the rhythm as ineffective and delivers a defibrillation. The rescuer need not be skilled in interpreting arrhythmias, although an experienced clinician can override the device and prevent the automatic discharge, if necessary.

Most episodes of sudden cardiac death are caused by ventricular fibrillation, which responds well to defibrillation. Thus, automatic defibrillators can have a significant impact on survival if they are readily available in shopping malls, fire departments, and anywhere people congregate. Emergency medical technicians and some firefighters are currently being trained to apply the device, and many emergency medical service systems are reviewing ways to expand its use to other first responders.

Automatic implantable cardioverter defibrillator

An automatic implantable cardioverter defibrillator (AICD) may be used for a patient who has experienced multiple episodes of ventricular tachycardia or ventricular fibrillation and who has not responded to antiarrhythmic drug therapy. The device is implanted in the patient's abdominal tissues, with electrodes attached to the heart's epicardial surface. When the AICD senses chaotic depolarizations or an unusually fast rate, it delivers a direct current of 25 to 30 joules to the heart—usually sufficient to convert the rhythm—and successive countershocks if the abnormal rhythm continues. (If a rescuer is performing CPR on a victim with an AICD and the device discharges, the shock may be perceptible but is not dangerous to the rescuer.) If the AICD does not effectively convert the rhythm, external defibrillation should be performed and routine ACLS protocols for the arrhythmia instituted.

Cardioversion

Cardioversion (or synchronized countershock) is a more appropriate intervention than defibrillation when the patient has a pulse. Synchronization prevents the electrical current from being delivered on the vulnerable phase of the T wave and inadvertently converting a rhythm with a pulse to a pulseless rhythm.

Rhythms treated with cardioversion include ventricular tachycardia (when the patient has a pulse and is unstable or has not responded to drug therapy), atrial fibrillation, atrial flutter, and unstable supraventricular tachycardia. Each of these rhythms has obvious QRS complexes. When the defibrillator is set for synchronization, the sensor recognizes the large depolarizations and discharges only on a QRS complex:

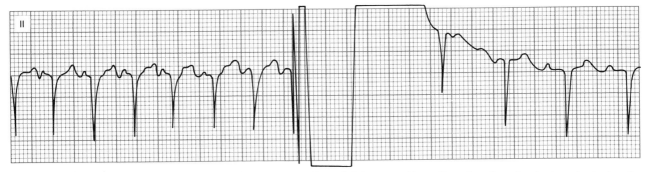

In this strip, the rapid reentry cycle characteristic of supraventricular tachycardia is interrupted by cardioversion. A synchronized countershock on the QRS complex produces the normal electrical conduction of a sinus rhythm.

Before charging the defibrillator, the operator should ensure that the machine is functioning. Most defibrillators display a light flash on each QRS complex to indicate proper sensing. If the light flashes do not appear, the operator may need to change to another lead in which the QRS amplitude is greater or increase the size of the QRS complex on the monitor.

Once the operator activates the synchronizer switch, the defibrillator will not discharge until the operator depresses the buttons and the defibrillator senses the QRS. Thus, if the patient's rhythm deteriorates to one without QRS complexes (ventricular fibrillation or asystole), the operator must turn off the synchronizer switch before attempting unsynchronized defibrillation.

Because cardioversion is used to interrupt an organized but rapid rhythm, energy levels lower than those used for defibrillation are usually effective: 50 to 100 joules for ventricular tachycardia and 75 to 100 joules for supraventricular tachycardia. Occasionally, lower levels (20 to 50 joules) may be used to convert atrial flutter or atrial fibrillation. If ineffective, the levels may be increased to those used for defibrillation.

Precordial thump

A precordial thump—a blow delivered with the side of the fist to the patient's midsternum—delivers a shock equivalent to a small amount of electrical current. The blow has been used to convert ventricular tachycardia and ventricular fibrillation and to stimulate a ventricular complex in complete heart block with ventricular standstill. Because the precordial thump does not have a high rate of effectiveness, only one thump is attempted and then only in a witnessed arrest. The procedure is taught in ACLS but is not recommended for use in BLS. A blow delivered incorrectly can injure the patient's ribs or internal organs. Occasionally, a thump may produce ventricular fibrillation or asystole. Not all institutions include a precordial thump as a part of their emergency protocol, so be well informed of your institution's policy.

Cardiac pacing

A pacemaker is an artificial pulse generator that delivers an electrical current directly to the heart via a catheter electrode to start a wave of depolarization. The most common pacemaker is a permanent implantable device, usually consisting of a small pulse generator with a lithium battery power source and an electrode inserted transvenously for delivering the electrical current to the heart's endocardial surface. The electrode is usually inserted through the subclavian vein and follows a venous pathway through the superior vena cava into the right side of the heart. The catheter has one or two electrodes near its tip, positioned so that it contacts the endocardium of the right ventricle.

A temporary pacemaker can be inserted transvenously via a largebore needle through which the catheter is threaded or applied to the epicardium during surgery. The newer external transcutaneous pacemakers have electrodes that are applied to the patient's chest. These pacemakers are valuable to prehospital intervention and for emergency use in the hospital, but they are inappropriate for longterm use. If continued pacing is necessary, the patient will need a transvenous pacemaker.

A pacemaker delivers a predetermined amount of electrical energy, measured in milliamperes. The operator determines the level by gradually increasing the current, once the electrode is in place, until capture (successful pacing with a pulse generator) is achieved and then increasing by 50% to 100% to overcome resistance. Capture is indicated on the ECG monitor by the spike or pacemaker discharge followed by a depolarization wave. If the atria are being paced, the pacer spike would be followed by a P wave:

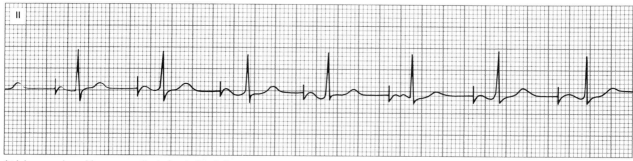

Atrial pacemaker with a pacer spike in front of each P wave.

If the ventricle is being paced, a QRS complex would follow the pacer spike:

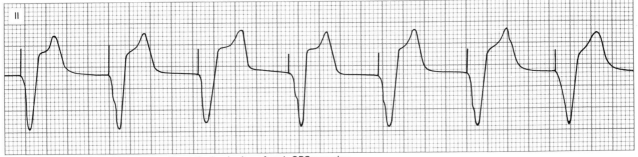

Ventricular pacemaker with a pacer spike at the beginning of each QRS complex.

The operator also determines the pacing rate by setting the pulse generator to discharge in a predetermined number of milliseconds. Most permanent pacemakers come from the manufacturer set at a rate of 72 discharges/minute (840 msec). This rate may be reprogrammed higher or lower by changing the milliseconds between discharges.

CARDIAC PACING RATES

Beats/minute	Milliseconds
40	1,500
50	1,200
60	1,000
70	857
72	840
80	750
90	667
100	600
110	545
120	500
150	400

Most pacemakers also sense spontaneous depolarization of a sufficient voltage and respond to this sensing with a preset mode. The mode may inhibit the pacemaker from firing or may be set to trigger firing in another site in the heart.

Pacemakers are classified by a generic letter code. The first letter of the code indicates the heart chamber being paced. The second

PACEMAKER IDENTIFICATION CODE

Chambers paced	Chambers sensed	Mode of response	Programmable functions	Antitachyarrhythmia functions
V = Ventricle	V = Ventricle	T = Triggered	P = Programmable (rate, output, or both)	P = Standard pacers technology
A = Atrium	A = Atrium	I = Inhibited	M = Multiprogrammable	S = Shock
S = Single chamber	S = Single chamber	D = Double	C = Communicating	D = Pacers and shock
D = Double chamber	D = Double chamber	O = None	R = Rate modulation	
O = None	O = None		O = None	

letter indicates the heart chamber being sensed (if the pacemaker does not sense, "O" is placed in this position). The third letter indicates the pacemaker's mode of response when it senses depolarization. For instance, if the pacemaker has an inhibited response ("I"), the pulse generator is prevented from firing and is reset to start counting the milliseconds again. Most common pacemakers are VVI (demand) pacemakers:

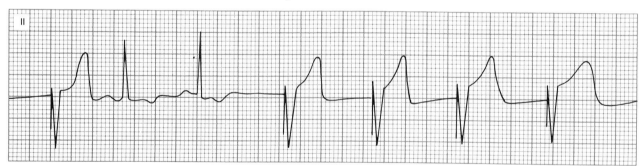

A VVI pacemaker paces in the ventricle (each pacer spike is followed by a QRS complex), senses in the ventricle (the second and third QRS complexes are sensed), and responds to sensing by inhibiting the pulse generator from firing (evidenced by lack of pacer spikes after the second QRS complex). The pacing rate is 840 msec, or 72 beats/minute. The pause rate is 840 msec, measured from the third beat (last intrinsic QRS complex) to the pacer spike of the next beat. Some pacemakers use the property of hysteresis, enabling the pause rate to be greater than the pacing rate.

An example of a pacemaker with a triggered response ("T") is a VAT pacemaker, which paces in the ventricle when it senses in the atria. The pacer spike always occurs a preset number of milliseconds after the atrial depolarization (P wave) is sensed. This ventricular pacing is essentially triggered by the sensing of a P wave or atrial depolarization:

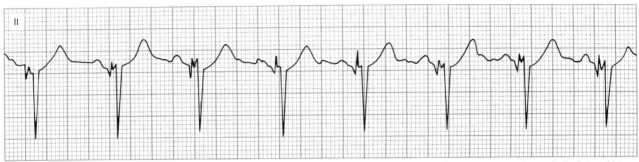

Atrial-triggered ventricular pacing. The pacemaker senses the P waves and responds by pacing the ventricles at a preset atrioventricular interval later. The pacer spikes are seen a fixed distance (number of milliseconds) after each P wave.

If the pacemaker does not sense, it would also not have a mode, so an "O" would appear in the third position. This type of pacemaker (VOO) fires at a fixed rate unrelated to any intrinsic cardiac activity.

Being used with greater frequency are reprogrammable pacemakers, which communicate with a reprogramming device that can change the pacing rate, milliamperes of electrical output, sensitivity, response modes, and other variables. The fourth letter of the pacemaker identification code indicates the programmable functions available. Many of these reprogrammable pacemakers have DDD capability — they can pace and sense in dual chambers (atrium and ventricle) and have a dual mode of response (inhibited and triggered):

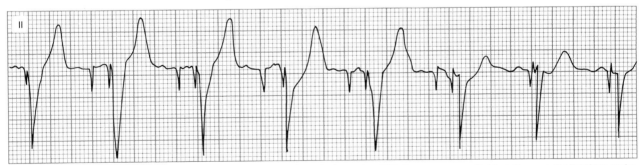

The first portion of the ECG strip above demonstrates both atrial and ventricular pacing. With the appearance of intrinsic P waves, the last three cycles show atrial-sensed, ventricular-paced beats.

The dual-chamber pacemaker is of particular value in the patient with poor pump function because it stimulates the atrium before the ventricles, approximating the normal sequence of events. DDD pacing usually increases cardiac output by restoring the atrial kick.

Some newer pacemakers also have an antitachycardia function. The fifth letter of the pacemaker identification code indicates the pacemaker response to a tachycardic rate.

Most pacemakers are used to augment a slow heart rate. Rhythms that might require a pacemaker include bradycardias that do not respond to drug therapy, such as sinus bradycardia, junctional escape rhythm, or second- or third-degree atrioventricular block. Pacing may also be indicated for frequent sinus arrests or sick sinus syndrome, ventricular tachycardia, or frequent ectopy. Pacing at a normal rate (70 to 80 beats/minute) may be used to treat torsades de pointes.

Pacemaker malfunctions

If a pacemaker's battery is weak, the pacing rate may decrease or the pacemaker may fail to discharge. Such a failure can be identified on an ECG monitor by the appearance of an unusually long pause. Intrinsic cardiac activity is absent, so pacemaker discharge would be expected but fails to occur. Lengthy or frequent pauses can reduce the heart rate, and the resulting decrease in cardiac output may cause the patient to seek treatment for syncope, dizziness, light-headedness, or weakness. The pacemaker's battery or pulse generator will need replacement.

Oversensing can occur if a pacemaker's sensing mechanism is set too high or if the pacemaker is exposed to certain types of electromagnetic interference. Under such conditions, the pacemaker might mistake noncardiac muscle activity, a high-voltage T wave, or an external current for cardiac depolarization. Such inappropriate sensing inhibits the pacemaker from firing, drastically lowering the pacing rate and producing long pauses on the ECG monitor:

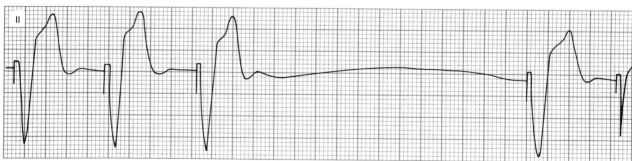

Oversensing or failure to fire.

Adjusting the sensitivity setting usually resolves oversensing or failure to fire. A pacemaker can also undersense or fail to sense depolarization. In such instances, pacer spikes occur inappropriately close to previous QRS complexes:

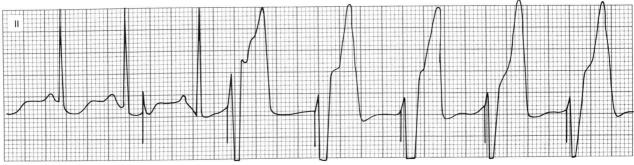

Undersensing or inappropriate pacing.

If one of the spikes fires during the vulnerable phase, R-on-T phenomenon and ventricular fibrillation can result. Undersensing can be caused by a dislodged electrode. Repositioning the patient or increasing the sensitivity setting may eliminate this problem.

A pacemaker may also fail to capture; that is, appropriate pacer spikes are not followed by depolarization. Possible causes include incorrect positioning of the pacer electrode, fracture of the pacer wire, and increased electrical resistance at the electrode site. If the patient has no intrinsic depolarizations, the rhythm would be asystole and should be treated accordingly. Increasing the milliamperes on a reprogrammable pacemaker may produce capture. If this proves ineffective, the pacemaker may need to be replaced.

Ventricular Fibrillation

Ventricular fibrillation (VF) is a life-threatening arrhythmia characterized by rapid and chaotic electrical activity, disorganized depolarization and repolarization of the ventricles, and a lack of effective mechanical contraction and cardiac output. The patient will require immediate basic life support.

The algorithm on the opposite page presents the established emergency treatment protocol for VF or pulseless ventricular tachycardia. Case studies incorporating the algorithm's interventions follow.

VENTRICULAR FIBRILLATION

This algorithm presents the emergency measures to take for a patient with ventricular fibrillation (VF) or pulseless ventricular tachycardia (VT). After each defibrillation, check the patient's pulse rate and rhythm. If the arrhythmia recurs after a transient conversion, repeat the joule level that produced the conversion. Intubate the patient earlier than shown, if possible. Some clinicians prefer administering lidocaine in 0.5 mg/kg boluses every 8 minutes to a total dosage of 3 mg/kg. Sodium bicarbonate is not recommended for routine cardiac arrest.

Witnessed cardiac arrest
▼
Check pulse. If absent,
administer precordial thump. ▶

Unwitnessed cardiac arrest
▼
Check pulse.
▼

If absent, initiate cardiopulmonary resuscitation (CPR) until a defibrillator is available. Check cardiac monitor to detect VF or VT.
▼
Defibrillate with 200 joules. If unsuccessful, defibrillate with 200 to 300 joules and, if still unsuccessful, with up to 360 joules.
▼
Check pulse. If absent, perform CPR. Establish I.V. line.
▼
Administer epinephrine 1:10,000, 0.5 to 1 mg I.V. push. Repeat dose every 5 minutes.
▼
Intubate as soon as possible.
▼
Defibrillate with up to 360 joules.
▼
Administer lidocaine, 1 mg/kg I.V. push.
▼
Defibrillate with up to 360 joules.
▼
Administer bretylium, 5 mg/kg I.V. push. (Consider administering sodium bicarbonate.)
▼
Defibrillate with up to 360 joules.
▼
Administer bretylium, 10 mg/kg I.V. push.
▼
Defibrillate with up to 360 joules.
▼
Repeat lidocaine or bretylium.
▼
Defibrillate with up to 360 joules.

Case study: Witnessed VF

After experiencing chest pain for 2 hours, Mrs. R. is admitted to the critical care unit for suspected myocardial infarction (MI). The patient, who weighs 154 lb (70 kg), had an anterior wall MI several years ago. Data on admission include these results: blood pressure, 110/60 mm Hg; heart rate, irregular; respiratory rate, 12 breaths/minute, with lungs clear to auscultation; creatine phosphokinase, 290 units/liter (normal value is less than 75 units/liter); CPK-MB, 13% (normal value is less than 10%).

Electrocardiogram (ECG) monitoring is initiated, revealing sinus bradycardia with frequent premature ventricular complexes and ST segment elevation in leads II, III, and aVF. The team leader administers 70 mg of lidocaine (Xylocaine) by I.V. bolus and orders a continuous I.V. drip.

ST segment elevation in leads II, III, and aVF and MB isoenzyme of 13% support the diagnosis of MI. Thus, the patient's ectopic beats must be treated aggressively.

While a team member is preparing the I.V. drip, the following rhythm appears on the monitor:

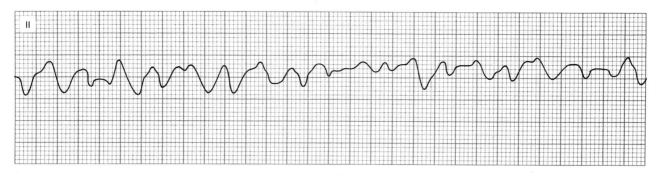

 Check pulse.
Administer precordial thump.
Check pulse.

Mrs. R. has no pulse. The team leader identifies the rhythm as VF and delivers a precordial thump. A team member immediately checks Mrs. R.'s pulse and rhythm.

Used only for a witnessed arrest, the precordial thump is a noninvasive and immediate way to shock the heart. The blow can depolarize a critical percentage of ventricular electrical system cells and allow normal depolarization. Because its effectiveness decreases considerably if not delivered immediately after onset of fibrillation, the precordial thump is not used for a nonwitnessed arrest. Immediately after the precordial thump is administered, a team member should check the patient's carotid pulse and rhythm on the monitor. Electrical rhythm may return without mechanical contraction, as evidenced by a rhythm on the monitor and a lack of pulse. (See Chapter 10, Electromechanical Dissociation, for a detailed discussion.)

Initiate CPR.

Mrs. R. remains pulseless and the arrhythmia continues, so the team initiates CPR.

Basic life support (BLS) is always important to begin and continue during advanced cardiac life support (ACLS). Advanced interventions will not sustain life without the basic interventions of maintaining oxygenation and circulation.

 Defibrillate with 200 joules.
Check pulse.

"Code Blue" is announced over the hospital paging system, and team members quickly bring the crash cart with defibrillator. A team member charges the defibrillator to 200 joules, and the team leader attempts defibrillation. The ECG monitor shows the following rhythm:

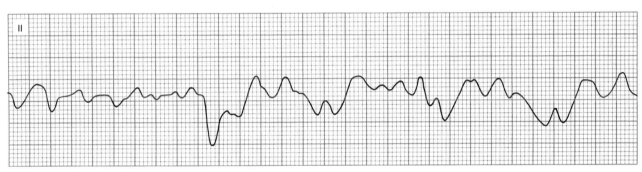

 Defibrillate with 200 to 300 joules.
Check pulse.

The rhythm is continued VF. Mrs. R. still has no pulse. The team leader defibrillates again, this time increasing the voltage to 300 joules.

The goal of defibrillation is to depolarize a critical percentage of cells and stimulate normal repolarization without damaging the cells. Thus, the recommended procedure is to begin with 200 joules and, if conversion to a normal rhythm does not occur, increase the electricity as outlined in the algorithm.

 Defibrillate with 200 to 300 joules.
Check pulse.

After the second defibrillation, Mrs. R.'s rhythm converts to sinus tachycardia for 3 seconds and then spontaneously reverts to VF. The team leader defibrillates again with 300 joules, and a team member rechecks Mrs. R.'s pulse and rhythm.

If VF recurs after a transient conversion to an organized rhythm, the next defibrillation should use the same amount of electricity as the previous one. Remember, the goal of defibrillation is to depolarize a critical percentage of cells without damaging them. A transient conversion to an organized rhythm may indicate that the correct amount of energy is being used. After each defibrillation, a team member should check the patient's pulse and rhythm for possible return of electrical rhythm without mechanical contraction.

Continue CPR.
Administer epinephrine.

While the team continues CPR, one of the team members administers 1 mg of epinephrine (Adrenalin) by I.V. push.

An I.V. line provides the most reliable absorption route for emergency cardiac medications during CPR. Epinephrine administration not only causes bronchodilation, thus promoting adequate ventilation and oxygenation, but also may help restore excitability of the heart and increase the effectiveness of defibrillation.

Initiate endotracheal intubation.

Next, the team initiates endotracheal intubation.

Endotracheal intubation should be accomplished as soon as possible after cardiac arrest. If the patient is already on a mechanical ventilator, the team should disconnect the ventilator and use a manual resuscitation bag connected to 100% oxygen. The bag resuscitator provides better ventilation and helps ensure adequate oxygenation during CPR.

Defibrillate with 360 joules.
Check pulse.

When Mrs. R. has been adequately ventilated, the team leader defibrillates her again, increasing the energy level to 360 joules.

Defibrillation is the definitive treatment for VF. The other interventions, principally endotracheal intubation and epinephrine administration, promote optimal oxygenation and permit pharmacologic support of cellular excitability, creating the best chances for successful defibrillation. Because an earlier attempt at 300 joules failed to convert the arrhythmia, the team leader appropriately increased the energy to 360 joules, the next recommended level in the algorithm.

After defibrillation, the following rhythm appears:

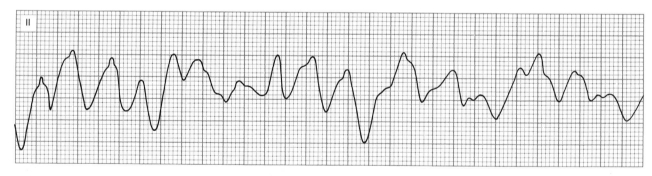

Administer lidocaine.

VF continues. Mrs. R. remains pulseless and unresponsive. The team leader administers 35 mg (0.5 mg/kg) of lidocaine.

Lidocaine decreases myocardial irritability and may improve the myocardial response to defibrillation. The initial dose for ventricular fibrillation is 1 mg/kg by I.V. bolus, followed by 0.5 mg/kg every 8 minutes to a maximum dose of 3 mg/kg. Note that lidocaine can be administered directly into an endotracheal tube if an I.V. line has not been established. If the endotracheal route is used, the lidocaine dosage is 100 mg followed by a 2- to 3-ml flush with sterile saline solution.

▼ Repeat epinephrine.

Five minutes have elapsed since the last epinephrine dose, so a team member administers another 1 mg by I.V. push.

Because epinephrine has a short duration of action, the dose is repeated every 5 minutes to increase cardiac contractility. The standard dose for VF is 0.5 to 1 mg of a 1:10,000 solution by I.V. bolus.

▼ Defibrillate with 360 joules.

The team leader again defibrillates Mrs. R. with 360 joules, and the following rhythm appears on the ECG monitor:

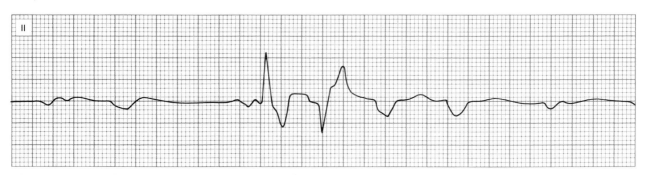

▼ Check pulse.

The rhythm shows continued VF. Mrs. R. remains pulseless. The team leader instructs a member to draw blood via the femoral artery for arterial blood gas (ABG) analysis.

ABG analysis helps determine whether ventilation is adequate and whether sodium bicarbonate administration is indicated to counteract the acidosis that occurs during a cardiac arrest. Acidosis results from lactic acid buildup secondary to anaerobic metabolism. Sodium bicarbonate used to be administered every 5 to 10 minutes for cardiac arrest to correct or prevent acidosis. However, the resulting alkalotic state can be as detrimental as acidosis, producing a paradoxical acidosis that further depresses the ischemic myocardium. Consequently, sodium bicarbonate administration is now guided by ABG values.

ABG analysis of Mrs. R. yields these results: pH, 7.29; Po_2, 74 mm Hg; Pco_2, 35 mm Hg; HCO_3, 11 mEq/liter; base deficit, -8. The team treats Mrs. R.'s acidosis (pH 7.29) by increasing the rate and depth of her respirations.

The slightly low Po_2 (normally 80 to 100 mm Hg) and the Pco_2 (normally 35 to 45 mm Hg) are acceptable. Acidosis has resulted from the low HCO_3 (normally 20 to 25 mEq/liter). Increasing the rate and depth of respirations should reduce the patient's acidosis and improve the Po$_2$ value.

Administer bretylium.

A team member assesses Mrs. R. for a carotid pulse and responsiveness, but her condition remains unchanged. The team leader orders 5 mg/kg of bretylium (Bretylol) by I.V. bolus.

Both lidocaine and bretylium are useful in treating VF that has not responded to defibrillation attempts. At this stage, some physicians choose to repeat doses of lidocaine rather than administer bretylium because the latter can lead to vasodilation and profound hypotension. Considering the patient's unresponsiveness to lidocaine, however, the team leader in this case opted for bretylium, which may prove more effective in treating the arrhythmia. *Note:* During a cardiac arrest, the team must continually reassess CPR and its effectiveness. Success of ACLS depends on adequate BLS.

Defibrillate with 360 joules.

The team again defibrillates Mrs. R. with 360 joules. On the ECG monitor, this rhythm appears:

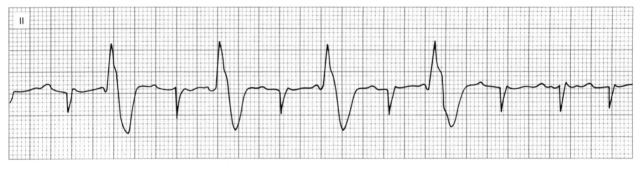

Check pulse.

The monitor shows a sinus rhythm with premature ventricular complexes. Mrs. R.'s pulse returns. Her blood pressure is 104/62 mm Hg. Although she remains unresponsive to verbal stimuli and touch, she responds appropriately to moderate pain. The team leader orders a bretylium infusion at 2 mg/minute.

The bretylium infusion is established to prevent cardiac irritability. (If defibrillation had been successful after lidocaine administration, a lidocaine infusion would have been ordered.) The patient's physician may also order electrolyte studies (hyperkalemia or hypokalemia can cause an arrhythmia) and an ABG analysis to confirm adequate oxygenation (hypoxia can cause myocardial irritability).

Case study: Unwitnessed VF

One evening, while writing out checks to pay the monthly bills, Mr. G., age 58, collapses at his desk and falls to the floor. His wife tries to revive him by shaking him and calling out his name, but he

Check pulse.
Initiate CPR.

does not respond. Unskilled in CPR, she dials 911 and asks the dispatcher to send help immediately. Several minutes later, paramedics arrive to find Mr. G. with no discernible pulse or blood pressure. They immediately initiate CPR.

As soon as rescuers determine that a person has no pulse, they must initiate and continue BLS until a pulse is palpable—an important guideline to remember during ACLS.

The paramedics apply electrodes to the man's chest and view the following rhythm on the ECG monitor:

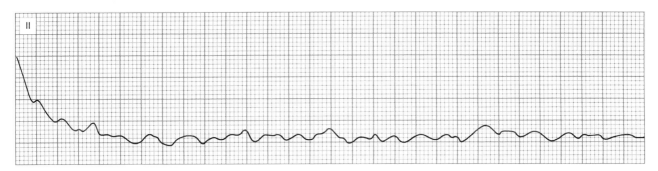

Defibrillate with 200 joules.

Mr. G. still has no pulse. The paramedics identify the rhythm as VF and defibrillate him with 200 joules.

VF is a disorganized rhythm marked by a lack of effective cardiac depolarization, mechanical contraction, and cardiac output. Defibrillation—the definitive treatment for this life-threatening arrhythmia—delivers electrical current to the myocardium to depolarize a critical mass of myocardial cells simultaneously. If successful, defibrillation induces organized repolarization and, subsequently, an organized, effective rhythm.

After defibrillation, the paramedics check Mr. G.'s rhythm on the monitor:

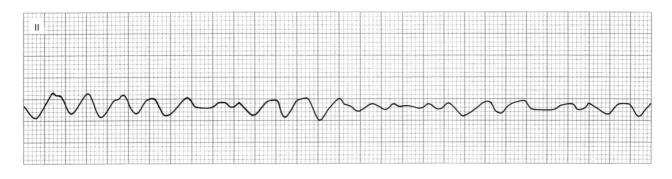

Check pulse.
Defibrillate with 200 to 300 joules.
Check pulse.
Defibrillate with 360 joules.

VF continues. Mr. G. remains pulseless and unresponsive. The paramedics continue BLS and defibrillate again, this time using 300 joules, but the rhythm does not change. They recheck Mr. G.'s pulse and defibrillate a third time, increasing the voltage to 360 joules.

Defibrillations of increasing force improve the odds of spontaneously depolarizing the myocardial cells and converting the arrhythmia to a normal rhythm. The recommended energy level for the first defibrillation is 200 joules; for the second, 200 to 300 joules; and for the third, 360 joules. Continuing BLS during cardiac arrest helps maintain circulation, perfusion, and ventilation (to prevent anoxic tissue damage).

Check pulse.
Continue CPR.
Establish I.V. line.
Administer epinephrine.

When the third defibrillation attempt fails, the paramedics decide to transport Mr. G. to the hospital. Continuing CPR en route, they also establish an I.V. line and administer 1 mg of epinephrine to Mr. G., flushing the drug with normal saline solution.

Drugs are absorbed more reliably and more rapidly when administered by the I.V. route. By stimulating beta receptors, epinephrine can increase cardiac excitability, enhance defibrillation attempts, and allow for subsequent effective mechanical contraction. Epinephrine also stimulates alpha receptors, which helps maintain tissue perfusion, produces peripheral vasoconstriction, and increases peripheral vascular resistance, aortic diastolic blood pressure, and coronary artery blood flow. Flushing epinephrine with normal saline solution helps ensure that the drug gets into the vein for absorption. (See Chapter 5, Pharmacologic Therapy, for more information on the effects of epinephrine.)

Initiate endotracheal intubation.

On arrival in the emergency department (ED), Mr. G. remains pulseless and unresponsive. The ED physician initiates endotracheal intubation.

Endotracheal intubation helps provide adequate oxygenation for the myocardium and has several advantages over bag-mask resuscitation. It isolates the airway, preventing aspiration; allows for suctioning of the trachea and bronchi; prevents wasted ventilation and gastric distention; and provides a route for administration of lidocaine, atropine, and epinephrine. Although bag-mouth breathing can be effective in preventing severe hypoxemia, maintaining an optimum mask fit is difficult. After intubation, rescuers should continue ventilation with the manual bag resuscitator and resume BLS.

The ED physician then directs the team to draw arterial and venous blood for analysis of arterial blood gases (ABGs) and electrolytes.

Rescuers may draw arterial and venous blood at this time, although this step is not included in the basic algorithm. Arterial blood is drawn to detect hypoxemia, acidosis, or alkalosis; venous blood, to detect abnormal levels of potassium, which can cause myocardial irritability.

ABG analysis yields these results: pH, 7.30; Po_2, 62 mm Hg; Pco_2, 58 mm Hg; HCO_3, 17 mEq/liter; base deficit, -6.

The patient's ABG values reveal hypoxemia and metabolic acidosis. The HCO_3 is low because cardiac arrest triggers anaerobic metabolism, which results in lactic acid accumulation and acidosis. Additionally, anaerobic metabolism does not produce energy as efficiently as aerobic metabolism.

Analysis of Mr. G.'s electrolyte levels yields these results: Na^+, 132; K^+, 3.0; Ca^{++}, 6.8; CO_2, 28; Cl^-, 103. The physician directs a team member to administer 40 mEq/liter of potassium by I.V. drip.

The most important values are potassium (K^-) and calcium (Ca^{++}). Recall that electricity within myocardial cells is generated through movement of electrolytes—specifically, sodium, potassium, and calcium—into and out of the cells (see Chapter 1, The Heart: Anatomy and Physiology). In this case, the patient's low potassium level may contribute to myocardial irritability and irregular electrical events, so potassium administration is advisable. Although the low calcium level may contribute to the myocardium's resistance to defibrillation, calcium administration may further reduce the potassium level, and the patient is not dangerously hypocalcemic. Use of calcium in cardiac arrest has not proved beneficial, and high levels may be detrimental.

After the potassium is administered, the ECG monitor displays the following rhythm:

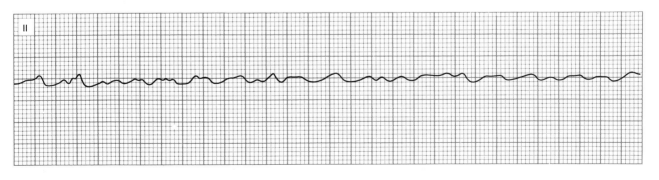

Check pulse.
Defibrillate with 360 joules.

Team members identify the rhythm as continued VF. Mr. G. remains pulseless and unresponsive, so a team member defibrillates him with 360 joules. The following rhythm appears on the ECG monitor:

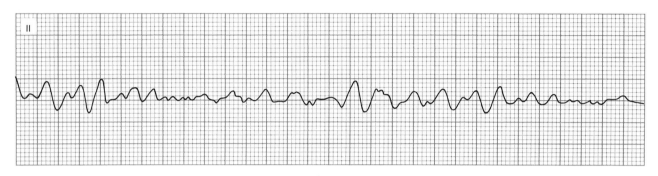

 Check pulse.
Administer epinephrine.

A team member rechecks Mr. G.'s pulse and rhythm. Ventricular fibrillation continues. The physician administers a 1-mg dose of epinephrine.

In cardiac arrest, epinephrine should be repeated every 5 minutes to optimize the conditions for defibrillation.

 Administer lidocaine.

After the epinephrine dose, the physician administers 75 mg of lidocaine by I.V. push.

Lidocaine, the drug of choice for managing ventricular irritability, may also improve the patient's response to defibrillation. The optimal dose is 1 mg/kg by I.V. bolus, although this can be approximated. Lidocaine is usually manufactured in prefilled syringes of 50 and 100 mg.

 Defibrillate with 360 joules.

A team member again defibrillates Mr. G. with 360 joules.

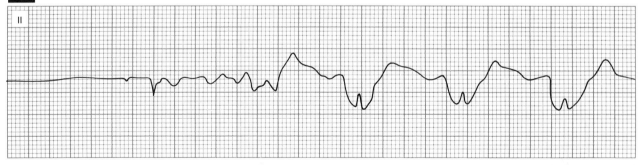

 Check pulse.
Continue CPR.
Administer bretylium.

Ventricular fibrillation continues. Mr. G. remains pulseless and unresponsive, so the team continues CPR efforts and the physician administers 350 mg of bretylium.

Although some rescuers would repeat the lidocaine dose at this point, others use bretylium when lidocaine fails to convert VF. The loading dose for bretylium is 5 mg/kg of body weight; the repeat dose is 10 mg/kg every 5 minutes. Bretylium is manufactured in prefilled syringes of 500 mg.

A team member again defibrillates Mr. G. with 360 joules. The following rhythm appears on the monitor:

▼ Defibrillate with 360 joules.

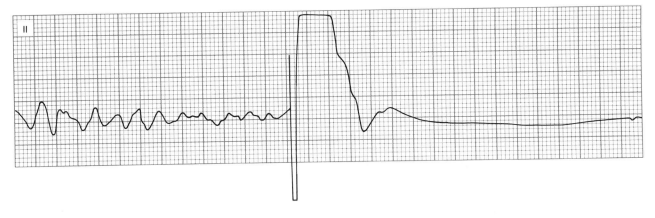

▼ Check pulse.

The team identifies the rhythm as asystole following defibrillation. Mr. G. still has no pulse and remains unresponsive to all life-saving interventions. The ED physician directs the team to terminate resuscitation efforts.

Study questions

Answers to study questions are on pages 98 and 99.
1. Working the night shift, you are checking your patients at 3 a.m. when you find Mr. R. pulseless and unresponsive. You press the bedside call button, and a "Code Blue" is announced over the loudspeaker. You and another nurse are performing CPR when the code team arrives. A team member quickly attaches monitor leads to the patient. The ECG monitor shows the following rhythm:

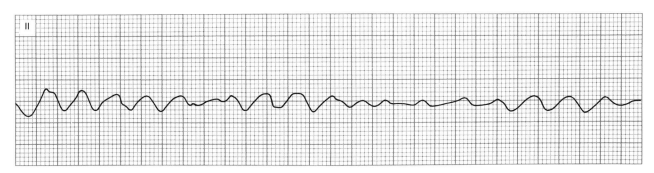

What should be the next intervention in this situation?

2. What is the next intervention?

3. VF continues. The patient remains pulseless and unresponsive. Describe the next five interventions.

4. Paramedics arrive at the ED with a patient in cardiac arrest. They report finding him unresponsive and without a pulse or respirations, placing him on a cardiac monitor (which revealed VF), and maintaining CPR throughout transfer. The ED physician defibrillates the patient with 200 joules and, when the patient remains pulseless, 300 and 360 joules. A nurse prepares an I.V. line and administers 1 mg of epinephrine by I.V. push. The ED physician then initiates endotracheal intubation, and ventilates the patient with 100% oxygen via a manual resuscitation bag. What should the next intervention be?

5. The patient's cardiac monitor displays the following rhythm:

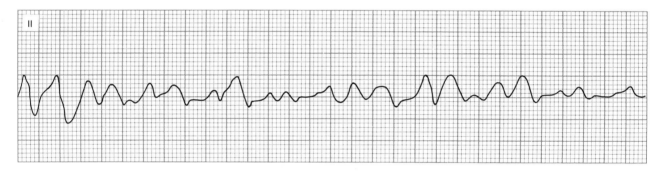

Describe the next intervention.

6. The patient still has no pulse. What is the next intervention?

7. Describe the next interventions.

8. A "Code Blue" is called in the intensive care unit. The patient, age 62, underwent coronary artery bypass graft surgery 3 days

ago. Because he had ectopy during surgery, 75 mg of lidocaine was administered by I.V. push and a continuous drip of 2 g of lidocaine in 500 ml of dextrose 5% in water (D_5W) was started at 2 mg/minute. Postoperative laboratory values include: Na^+, 137 mEq/liter (normal, 136 to 145 mEq/liter); K^+, 2.9 mEq/liter (normal, 3.5 to 5.0 mEq/liter); Cl^-, 98 mEq/liter (normal, 98 to 106 mEq/liter); Ca^{++}, 7.9 mg/dl (normal, 9 to 11 mg/dl); Hgb, 10.4 g/dl (normal mean, 15 g/dl); Hct, 30.5% (normal mean, 43%); pH, 7.48; Po_2, 101; Pco_2, 32; HCO_3, 26; base excess, 1; O_2 saturation, 98%. The patient's ECG rhythm is:

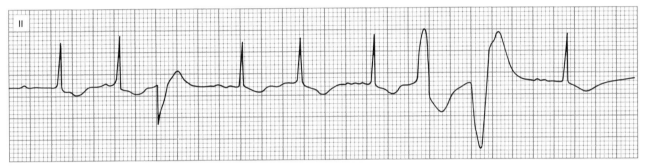

The physician orders 40 mEq of potassium to be administered by I.V. drip, mixed in 100 ml of D_5W. After the potassium administration, the patient's rhythm converts to the following:

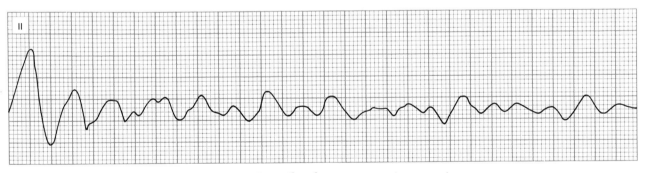

Describe the necessary interventions.

Answers to study questions

1. Defibrillate at 200 joules. As soon as the crash cart arrives, the team should attempt defibrillation for VF.

2. Check for pulse and return of normal rhythm.

3. The next five interventions would be:

   - Defibrillate at 200 to 300 joules and at 360 joules.

   - Continue CPR if the patient remains pulseless.

   - Establish an I.V. line.

   - Administer 1 mg of epinephrine by I.V. push.

   - Initiate endotracheal intubation.

4. Defibrillate with 360 joules. Defibrillation is the definitive treatment for VF. After epinephrine administration to increase alpha and beta stimulation to the heart and vascular system, defibrillate again.

5. Always check for a pulse after a defibrillation attempt.

6. Administer 1 mg/kg of lidocaine by I.V. push (to decrease myocardial irritability and improve the chances of successful defibrillation).

7. Defibrillate again at 360 joules, and repeat drug doses as indicated. Always defibrillate after administering a drug, because drug therapy improves the chances of successful defibrillation. Bretylium 5 mg/kg by I.V. push may be given if lidocaine proves ineffective. Because the drugs have short half-lives, lidocaine (0.5 mg/kg) is repeated every 8 minutes up to a maximum dose of 3 mg/kg, and bretylium (10 mg/kg) is repeated every 15 to 30 minutes up to a maximum dose of 30 mg/kg.

8. For witnessed VF, first deliver a precordial thump to the patient's chest and check for a pulse; then follow, as needed, with these interventions:

• Defibrillate at 200 joules. (Since the patient is in an intensive care unit, a defibrillator should be readily available. If a defibrillator cannot be obtained in less than 1 minute, initiate CPR.)

• If the rhythm does not change, defibrillate again at 200 to 300 joules and then at 360 joules.

• If the patient continues in VF, begin BLS to maintain artificial circulation and oxygenation. The postoperative patient is probably intubated, so use a manual resuscitation bag to provide adequate oxygenation. With an I.V. line already in place, administer epinephrine to improve the chances of successful defibrillation. Additionally, the physician would increase the dosage of the lidocaine drip to reduce myocardial irritability and promote conversion to a normal rhythm.

8

Ventricular Tachycardia

Because of its rapid rate and the resultant loss of atrial-ventricular synchrony, ventricular tachycardia (VT) usually compromises cardiac output. This chapter focuses on the patient requiring treatment for sustained episodes. If the patient is pulseless, follow the algorithm for ventricular fibrillation on page 85. For nonsustained tachycardia, treat the patient according to the algorithm for ventricular ectopy on page 167.

The algorithm on the opposite page presents the established emergency treatment protocol for sustained VT. Case studies incorporating the algorithm's interventions follow.

SUSTAINED VENTRICULAR TACHYCARDIA

This algorithm presents the emergency measures to take for a patient with sustained ventricular tachycardia (VT). Most interventions depend on whether the patient is stable or unstable. An unstable patient will have chest pain, dyspnea, hypotension, congestive heart failure, ischemia, or myocardial infarction. Consider using a precordial thump before cardioversion in a conscious unstable patient without hypotension or pulmonary edema. If cardioversion alone is unsuccessful in a patient who is hypotensive or unconscious or who has pulmonary edema, administer lidocaine (Xylocaine) and then bretylium (Bretylol). For other patients, administer lidocaine, procainamide (Pronestyl), or bretylium. Once VT resolves, infuse the antiarrhythmic drug that aided resolution.

No pulse	*Pulse present*	
▼	▼	▼
Treat as ventricular fibrillation.	Stable patient	Unstable patient
	▼	▼
	Administer oxygen. Establish I.V. line.	Administer oxygen. Consider sedation. Establish I.V. line.
	▼	▼
	Administer lidocaine, 1 mg/kg (then 0.5 mg/kg every 8 minutes until VT resolves or total dose of 3 mg/kg is reached).	Institute cardioversion with 50 joules. If the first attempt is unsuccessful, repeat at 100, 200, and 360 joules.
	▼	▼
	Administer procainamide 20 mg/minute until VT resolves or total dose of 1,000 mg is reached.	If VT recurs, administer lidocaine and institute cardioversion again, using the previous successful energy level. Then administer procainamide or bretylium.
	▼	
	Institute cardioversion if patient becomes unstable.	

Case study: Pulseless VT

Mr. M., age 42, is admitted to the emergency department (ED) with substernal chest pain and an ache radiating to his left jaw that began 6 hours ago. He appears diaphoretic and apprehensive. The patient, who weighs about 200 lb (90 kg), has no history of cardiac problems. Data on admission include the following: blood pressure, 140/86 mm Hg; heart rate, irregular; respiratory rate, 22 breaths/ minute, with lungs clear on auscultation. ED staff members draw blood for creatine phosphokinase (CPK) and lactic dehydrogenase (LDH) isoenzyme analysis, start an I.V. infusion of 5% dextrose in water (D_5W) at a keep-vein-open rate, and administer oxygen via nasal cannula at 4 liters/minute. They also place Mr. M. on a cardiac monitor, which shows the following rhythm:

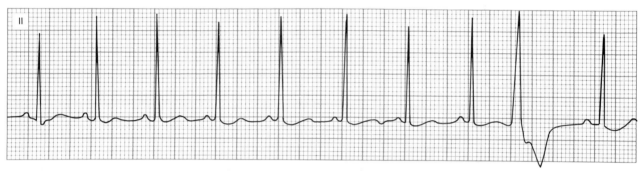

Staff members recognize the rhythm as sinus tachycardia with premature ventricular complexes (PVCs). Before they can inter-vene, however, Mr. M. suddenly gasps, and the monitor displays this rhythm:

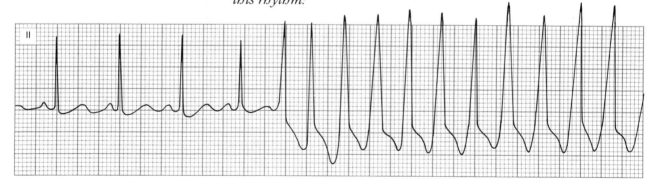

No pulse. Treat as ventricular fibrillation (see page 85).

Mr. M. does not respond when staff members call his name and gently shake him. The ED physician instantly recognizes the change to VT and delivers a precordial thump to Mr. M.'s chest.

The precordial thump can be used for witnessed VT in an unrespon-sive patient. The blow may successfully convert the rhythm, although it may also have no effect or cause the rhythm to deteriorate to ventricular fibrillation (VF) or asystole.

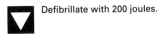 Defibrillate with 200 joules.

Mr. M. remains pulseless and unresponsive. A staff member retrieves the crash cart and defibrillates Mr. M. with 200 joules.

In pulseless VT, the patient lacks effective cardiac output, and the myocardium becomes even more ischemic with lack of circulation. Thus, the health care team must work swiftly to reverse the problem, either by circulating the blood artificially with cardiopulmonary resuscitation (CPR) or by establishing an effective rhythm. Interventions for pulseless VT are the same as for VF (see the algorithm for VF on page 85). Immediate defibrillation has the greatest likelihood of success. If a defibrillator is not immediately available, staff members should begin CPR.

After the first defibrillation attempt, the staff view this rhythm on the monitor:

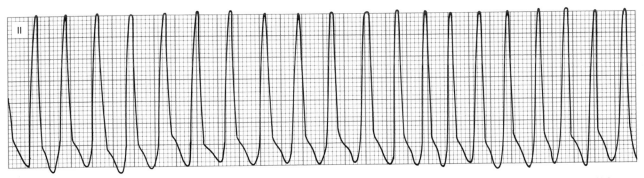

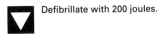 Defibrillate with 300 joules.

Ventricular tachycardia continues uninterrupted. Mr. M. still has no pulse, so the team leader attempts defibrillation again, this time using 300 joules.

The energy level for a second defibrillation is not always increased from the initial 200 joules used (the recommended level for a second attempt is 200 to 300). The first defibrillation lowers the electrical resistance of the chest wall for the second. Because the patient is a fairly large man, the team leader decided to increase the energy level to the maximum recommended.

The second defibrillation converts Mr. M.'s rhythm to the following:

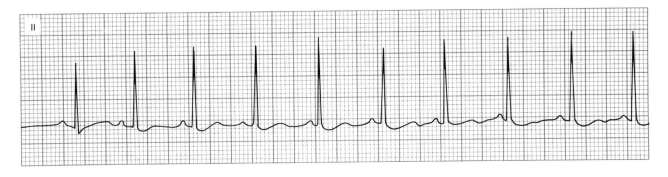

Administer lidocaine.

A normal sinus rhythm returns. Mr. M.'s pulse is weak but regular at 100 beats/minute. His blood pressure is 96/50 mm Hg. He is awake and moaning. The physician orders 90 mg of lidocaine (Xylocaine) by I.V. bolus.

Although a normal rhythm has been restored, the physician orders lidocaine to prevent recurrence of ventricular ectopy. Lidocaine effectively raises the threshold for VF and sufficiently alters electrophysiology to inhibit reentry PVCs or VT.

The physician also orders a lidocaine drip of 2 mg/minute. About 10 minutes later, Mr. M.'s blood pressure is 100/62 mm Hg. The electrocardiogram (ECG) monitor displays the following rhythm:

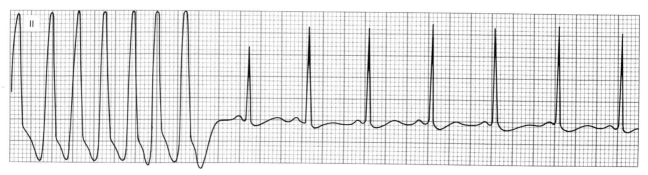

Mr. M. experiences a burst of nonsustained VT. The physician orders 45 mg of lidocaine by I.V. bolus.

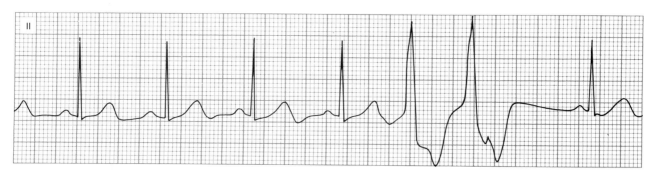

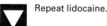 Repeat lidocaine.

Eight minutes later, ventricular ectopy (indicated by paired PVCs) is still evident on the monitor. The physician orders another 45 mg of lidocaine by I.V. bolus and increases the lidocaine drip to 3 mg/ minute.

Lidocaine boluses are repeated every 8 to 10 minutes (every 2 to 5 minutes for PVCs) until ventricular ectopy subsides or the maximum total dose of 3 mg/kg is reached. If ectopy ceases, a lidocaine drip is started to maintain that effective therapeutic blood level. If ectopy recurs, additional boluses are administered at 0.5 mg/kg. The drip dose is increased proportionally to the amount of additional boluses to maintain the new blood level.

Mr. M.'s monitor now displays this rhythm:

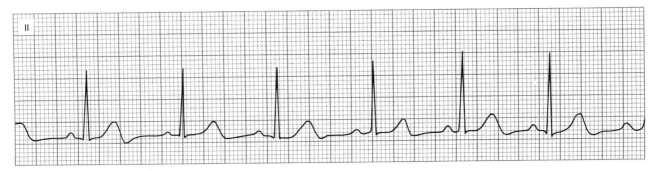

The monitor shows sinus rhythm without ectopy. Mr. M. is alert and responsive. Oxygen is being administered at 4 liters/minute. A nurse readies a second I.V. line before staff members transport him to the coronary care unit (CCU) for further observation and treatment.

Case study: Stable VT

Mrs. K., age 64, has just finished lunch and is sitting in a chair next to her bed in the CCU. Admitted 2 days ago with an inferior wall myocardial infarction (MI), she is receiving oxygen via a nasal cannula at 3 liters/minute. Mrs. K. has an I.V. heparin lock and is connected to an ECG monitor, which shows the following rhythm:

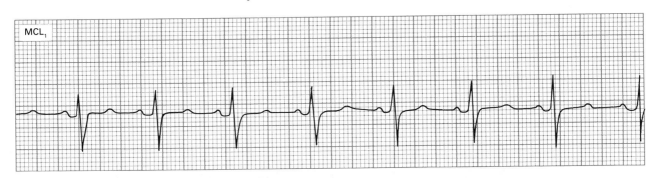

Mrs K. has a normal sinus rhythm. She has been pain-free for 7 hours and is in a talkative mood, much as she was just before lunch when a nurse checked her vital signs: blood pressure, 110/76

mm Hg; heart rate, 90 beats/minute; respiratory rate, 20 breaths/ minute, with basilar rales that clear with coughing. Now, however, a faster rhythm begins to appear on the monitor, although Mrs. K. continues to talk to the nurse in her room, apparently unaware of the rhythm change:

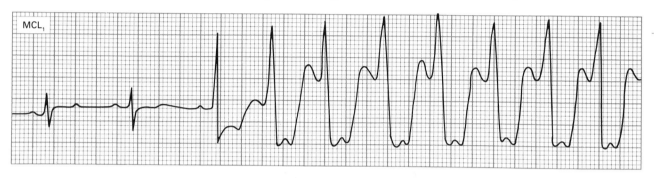

The nurse recognizes the rhythm as VT and rechecks Mrs. K.'s blood pressure (100/70 mm Hg) and heart rate (115 beats/ minute).

A patient who remains conscious and continues to carry on a conversation must be maintaining cardiac output. Thus, a nurse would have time to check the patient's vital signs and reassess the situation.

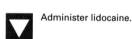

Administer lidocaine.

The nurse increases the oxygen level to 6 liters/minute and, according to protocol, administers 50 mg of lidocaine by I.V. bolus via the heparin lock and an I.V. drip of D_5W at a keep-vein-open rate. The nurse then notifies Mrs. K.'s physician of the rhythm.

Because the patient's rhythm and vital signs are stable, aggressive interventions are contraindicated. A precordial thump or defibrillation may produce an even faster rate, possibly deteriorating to VF.

Repeat lidocaine.

VT continues, but Mrs. K. remains alert and talkative, asking about her medication and the hanging of the I.V. bottle. Team members arrive and administer 25 mg of lidocaine by I.V. bolus. After reassuring Mrs. K., the nurse rechecks her blood pressure (102/70 mm Hg). The team obtains a 12-lead ECG:

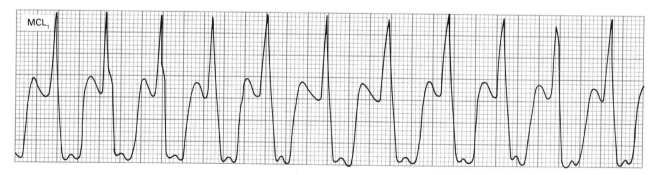

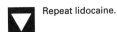

Repeat lidocaine.

The 12-lead ECG enables the physician to verify VT, showing atrioventricular (AV) dissociation with occasional P waves at a slower rate, left axis deviation, and a QRS complex of 0.14 to 0.16 second. About 8 minutes have elapsed since the last dose, so a team member administers another 25 mg of lidocaine by I.V. bolus.

In a stable patient, VT can be verified on a 12-lead ECG to rule out a wide complex supraventricular tachycardia. If the patient is unstable or pulseless, one would not take the time to obtain a 12-lead ECG but would immediately institute cardioversion or defibrillate the patient. Indicators for VT include QRS complexes greater than 0.14 second, AV dissociation, left axis deviation, monophasic complexes, precordial concordance (QRS complexes in chest leads are either all positive or all negative), and fusion beats.

Repeat lidocaine.
Administer procainamide.

About 10 minutes later, the team leader administers another 25 mg of lidocaine, without a change in Mrs. K.'s rhythm, and then draws blood for serum electrolyte studies. The nurse rechecks Mrs. K.'s blood pressure (102/72 mm Hg) and heart rate (110 beats/ minute). Then the leader administers 100 mg of procainamide (Pronestyl) I.V. over 5 minutes. The ECG monitor shows the rhythm convert to the following:

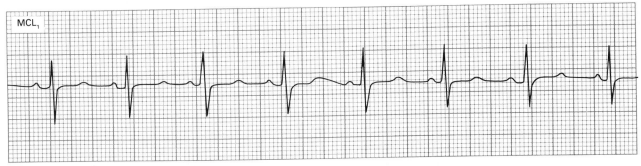

MCL₁

Normal sinus rhythm returns. Mrs. K.'s blood pressure is 100/70 mm Hg. A team member starts a procainamide drip at 2 mg/ minute.

If lidocaine at the maximum dosage is unsuccessful, the recommended intervention is to switch to procainamide. Follow the initial dose of procainamide, if unsuccessful, with additional doses at 20 mg/minute until a sinus rhythm returns, the patient becomes hypotensive, or the QRS complex widens by 50% or more. Once sinus rhythm returns, start an I.V. drip to maintain the therapeutic blood level. In the case study, a procainamide drip was used because lidocaine had not been successful in achieving this level. Subsequently, the team members would continue to investigate the cause of the patient's VT by reviewing her laboratory work and monitoring any rhythm changes that occur with patient activity.

Case study: Unstable VT

Mr. J., age 78, is brought to the ED by his daughter, who provides history-taking information for her Spanish-speaking father. She states that Mr. J. has been feeling bad for the last 24 hours. He clutches his left shoulder when placed on the gurney. Staff members administer oxygen via nasal cannula at 3 liters/minute, apply chest electrodes, and start an I.V. infusion of D₅W.

Mr. J. weighs about 132 lb (60 kg). Data on admission include a blood pressure of 128/82 mm Hg; a heart rate of 128 beats/ minute, with sinus tachycardia evident on the ECG monitor; and a respiratory rate of 28 breaths/minute, with rales in both lung bases.

As Mr. J. begins coughing, his rhythm on the monitor changes:

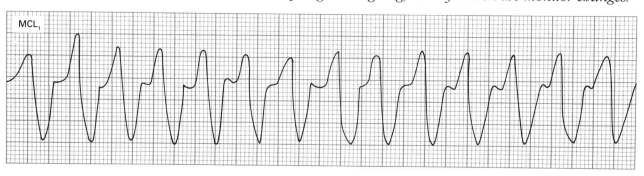

Team members recognize the rhythm as VT. Mr. J.'s pulse seems weaker than before. A team member checks his blood pressure, which has dropped to 86/50 mm Hg. He says he feels light-headed. The team leader decides to begin cardioversion (synchronized countershock).

The patient's condition is unstable. Congestion, light-headedness, decreased blood pressure, and a weaker pulse rate indicate that the patient's cardiac output is inadequate.

While a nurse escorts Mr. J.'s daughter to the waiting room to explain cardioversion to her, the team leader reviews the procedure with Mr. J., carefully explaining in both English and Spanish. He then administers 5 mg of diazepam (Valium) I.V. as another member prepares the defibrillator for synchronization. The leader then attempts cardioversion at 50 joules.

VT is an organized rhythm, so the countershock is synchronized to be delivered on the R wave of the QRS complex. Synchronization

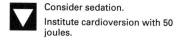

Consider sedation.
Institute cardioversion with 50 joules.

prevents inadvertent discharge on the T wave, which could cause the rhythm to deteriorate to VF. A relatively low energy level is used initially because higher levels are rarely necessary to convert VT.

 Repeat cardioversion at 100 joules.

Mr. J.'s rhythm and pulse remain unchanged, so the team leader attempts cardioversion again, this time at 100 joules. Mr. J.'s rhythm converts to the following:

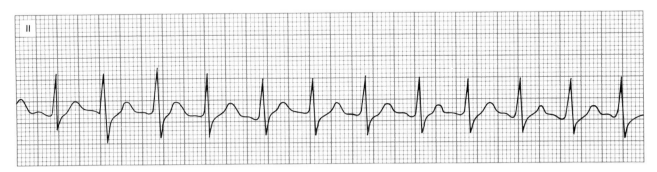

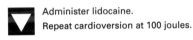 Administer lidocaine.
Repeat cardioversion at 100 joules.

Team members identify the rhythm as sinus tachycardia. Mr. J.'s pulse rate appears to be stronger. A team member rechecks his blood pressure, which has improved to 118/80 mm Hg. In a few moments, however, the rhythm reverts to VT. Mr. J. seems groggy but still responds to verbal stimuli and his pulse rate remains stable. The team leader administers 60 mg of lidocaine by I.V. bolus and repeats cardioversion at 100 joules.

Although low energy levels usually convert VT, the recurrence rate is fairly high. In such instances, the recommended procedure is to repeat the energy level that successfully converted the rhythm earlier.

Mr. J.'s rhythm converts to sinus tachycardia. A team member starts an I.V. infusion of lidocaine at 2 mg/minute.

Antiarrhythmic agents, such as lidocaine, help stabilize the patient, permitting later transfer to the intensive care unit for further observation and treatment.

Case study: Torsades de pointes

Mrs. W., age 58, is in the transitional care unit for episodes of palpitations accompanied by brief light-headedness. She has an I.V. heparin lock in place. Her history includes an anterolateral MI, premature atrial complexes, and PVCs. For the past 6 months, Mrs. W. has been taking maintenance doses of procainamide (500 mg every 6 hours). Only moments ago, a nurse checked her vital signs: blood pressure, 118/84 mm Hg; heart rate, 70 beats/minute; respiratory rate, 14 breaths/minute. Laboratory results obtained earlier revealed a total CPK of 160 and a CPK-MB of 0.8%.

During the last 6 hours, Mrs. W.'s monitor has continued to show sinus rhythm, but now the rate increases:

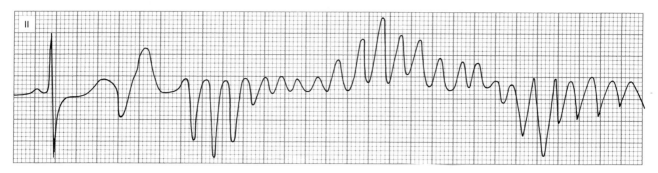

The rhythm is torsades de pointes, a form of VT.

Torsades de pointes does not usually respond to interventions routinely used for nonsustained episodes of VT. For example, lidocaine usually does not convert the rhythm or prevent a recurrence.

Mrs. W. converts spontaneously out of the rhythm but over the next 20 minutes has several more episodes, none lasting more than 6 seconds. Each time, she converts spontaneously. During the episodes, the nurse cannot palpate her pulse, although a strong pulse resumes on conversion. The ECG monitor shows a prolonged QT interval, a hallmark of torsades de pointes:

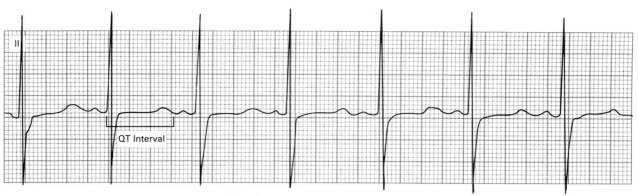

The physician orders blood drawn to determine serum electrolyte levels and a blood level of procainamide. Based on the results, he discontinues the procainamide.

Torsades de pointes can be caused by high blood levels of Class IA antiarrhythmics or by electrolyte imbalances, such as hypokalemia or hypomagnesemia. Patients usually have nonsustained episodes. If the rhythm is sustained, defibrillation may be attempted. Cardiac pacing at a normal rate (70 to 80 beats/minute) is sometimes used to convert the rhythm or to control repetitive episodes. Despite its side effects, isoproterenol (Isuprel) may be administered to shorten the QT interval and prevent the rhythm. Magnesium sulfate and bretylium are optional treatments.

Study questions

Answers to study questions are on page 113.

1. Mr. B., who weighs about 155 lb (70 kg), is a patient in the CCU where you work. Over the last several minutes, an increasing number of PVCs have accompanied his sinus rhythm, and now you note the following rhythm on the ECG monitor:

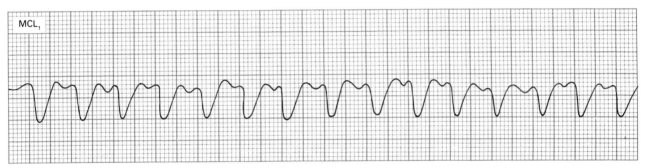

Interpret the rhythm.

2. You assess Mr. B., checking his pulse and blood pressure (108/ 70 mm Hg). He is alert and responsive. Oxygen is already being administered at 4 liters/minute via nasal cannula. Describe the next intervention.

3. The rhythm continues, and Mr. B.'s vital signs remain unchanged for the next 8 minutes. What is the next intervention?

4. After the physician administers three boluses of lidocaine (total dose 140 mg), Mr. B.'s rhythm converts to the following:

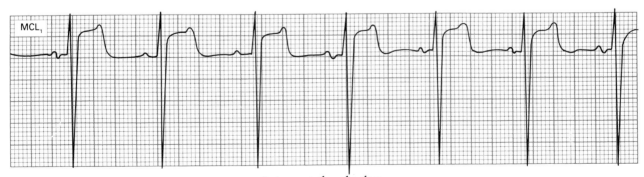

Interpret the rhythm.

5. You recheck Mr. B.'s blood pressure (130/80 mm Hg) and heart rate (70 beats/minute). Describe three appropriate interventions to maintain his rhythm.

6. Mr. M., who weighs about 175 lb (80 kg), is unresponsive when you enter his room to check him. After calling a code, you lower the head of the bed and open his airway, using a chin-lift technique, to assess his breathing—no spontaneous ventilations. Using the mask at the bedside, you ventilate Mr. M. with two breaths given over 1.5 seconds each and assess for a pulse but cannot detect one. As you begin cardiac compressions, the code team arrives with the crash cart. Using the "quick look" paddles, the team observes the following rhythm:

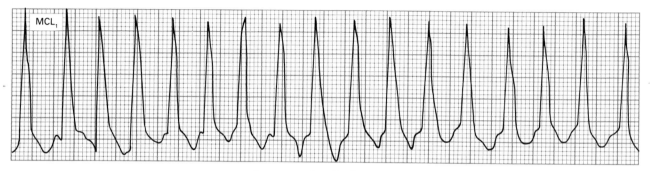

Interpret the rhythm.

7. What should be the next intervention?

8. Describe the next intervention.

9. Mr. M. remains pulseless and unresponsive. Describe the next four interventions.

10. Mr. M.'s condition remains unchanged, so the next step would be to maintain circulation. Describe how to accomplish this.

11. The next step should enhance the myocardial environment to facilitate defibrillation. Describe the next three steps.

12. After the above steps are taken, Mr. M. is defibrillated at 360 joules. The following rhythm appears on the monitor:

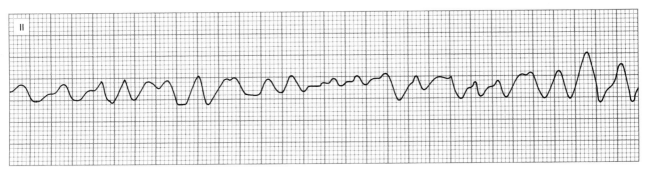

Interpret the rhythm.

13. Mr. M. remains pulseless and unresponsive. Describe the next intervention.

14. The code team continues CPR to circulate the drug. What is the next appropriate intervention?

Answers to study questions

1. VT (stable)

2. Administer 70 mg of lidocaine by I.V. bolus.

3. Administer 35 mg of lidocaine by I.V. bolus. (This may be repeated every 8 to 10 minutes, up to a total dose of 3 mg/kg, or 210 mg for this patient.)

4. Sinus rhythm

5. Start a lidocaine drip at 3 mg/minute, continue oxygen, and monitor vital signs and rhythm.

6. VT (pulseless)

7. Defibrillate with 200 joules.

8. Check for pulse and check monitor.

9. Defibrillate with 200 to 300 joules. Recheck the pulse and rhythm. If VT persists, defibrillate with 360 joules. Recheck the pulse and rhythm.

10. Perform CPR.

11. Establish an I.V. line. Administer epinephrine, 0.5 to 1 mg of a 1:10,000 solution I.V. Initiate endotracheal intubation.

12. VF

13. Administer lidocaine 1 mg/kg, which may be repeated in 5 to 8 minutes at 5 mg/kg up to a total dose of 3 mg/kg.

14. Defibrillate with 360 joules.

9 Ventricular Asystole

Ventricular asystole, also called ventricular or cardiac standstill, is the absence of electrical or mechanical activity in the myocardium. Because asystole usually is associated with prolonged cardiac arrest or end-stage cardiac dysfunction, the prognosis for a patient with asystole is poor. Nursing care focuses on basic life support (BLS) and on advanced cardiac life support (ACLS) techniques until electrical or mechanical function is restored.

The algorithm on the opposite page presents the established emergency treatment protocol for asystole. Case studies incorporating the algorithm's interventions follow.

ALGORITHM

VENTRICULAR ASYSTOLE

This algorithm presents the emergency measures to take for a patient with ventricular asystole. Because ventricular fibrillation (VF) can mimic asystole in some leads, you should confirm asystole in at least two leads. If uncertain whether the rhythm is asystole or fine VF, treat the rhythm as though it were VF and defibrillate the patient.

Initiate CPR.

Establish an I.V. line.

Administer epinephrine, 1:10,000, 0.5 to 1 mg I.V. push.
(Repeat the dose every 5 minutes.)

Insert endotracheal tube as soon as possible.

Administer atropine, 1 mg I.V. push.
(Repeat the dose in 5 minutes.)

Consider administering sodium bicarbonate.
(Repeat half of original dose every 10 minutes.)

Consider initiating pacemaker therapy.

Case study: Asystole resulting from heart block

Mr. P., age 52, is in the coronary care unit awaiting pacemaker insertion for a third-degree heart block. The bedside electrocardiogram (ECG) monitor shows the following rhythm:

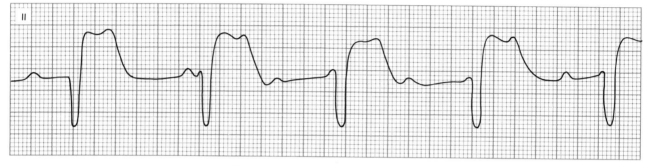

This rhythm strip indicates third-degree heart block with a ventricular pacer. In third-degree heart block, the atria and the ventricles are depolarized and contract independently. (See Chapter 4, Arrhythmia Interpretation, for a detailed discussion.)

Suddenly, the rhythm on Mr. P.'s bedside monitor changes:

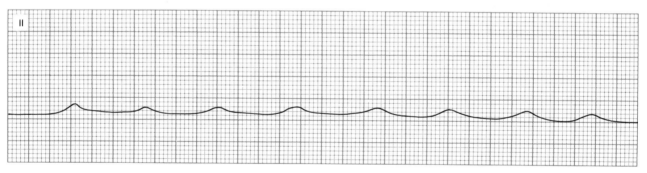

A nurse gently shakes Mr. P. and loudly calls out his name, but he doesn't respond. After checking the rhythm in another lead to verify asystole, the nurse calls for help. Mr. P. has no pulse.

Always check the patient's responsiveness before initiating emergency treatment measures. Verifying asystole in two leads is also important because fine ventricular fibrillation, which can be treated with defibrillation, can mimic asystole in some leads.

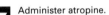

Initiate CPR.

The nurse verifies asystole and begins cardiopulmonary resuscitation (CPR).

Once asystole is confirmed, BLS is necessary to maintain the patient's ventilation and circulation. Although the algorithm does not specify this, you should always administer oxygen at 100% or 1.0 FIO_2 during CPR.

Administer epinephrine.

Since Mr. P. already has an I.V. line in place, a code team member administers 1 mg of epinephrine 1:10,000 by I.V. push.

Epinephrine, a catecholamine, stimulates the myocardium directly through the sympathetic nervous system.

Initiate endotracheal intubation.

The team leader inserts a 7-mm endotracheal tube, and other team members continue to ventilate Mr. P. with a manual resuscitation bag at 100% O_2.

A patient with asystole should be intubated as quickly as possible to provide better ventilation. As the algorithm's sequence suggests, however, CPR and epinephrine administration are higher priorities if the patient is being ventilated adequately with a resuscitation bag and mask.

Administer atropine.

One of the code team members checks Mr. P.'s pulse during a 5-second break in CPR. Mr. P. still has no pulse, so the team continues CPR. A nurse draws blood for arterial blood gas (ABG) analysis, and the team leader administers 1 mg of atropine by I.V. push.

During CPR, the patient should be checked at least every 5 minutes for a return of pulse. ABG analysis determines acid-base balance and adequacy of ventilation. Atropine, a parasympatholytic drug, increases sinus node automaticity and atrioventricular (AV) conduction. The drug is included in the algorithm for asystole although its beneficial effects are unproven. Asystolic cardiac arrest is usually fatal regardless of the therapy.

The ABG report on Mr. P. reveals these values: pH, 7.30; Pao_2, 88 mm Hg; $Paco_2$, 55 mm Hg; and HCO_3, 20 mEq/liter. The code team leader orders an increase in the rate and depth of ventilations.

The ABG results indicate that the patient has both metabolic and respiratory acidosis, a common complication in cardiac arrest. Increasing the rate and depth of ventilations should correct the problem. Note that administration of sodium bicarbonate is not recommended for routine cardiac arrest but may be considered later. If the patient had a severe acidosis, 1 mEq/kg of sodium bicarbonate would be an appropriate dose.

Mr. P.'s rhythm appears as follows:

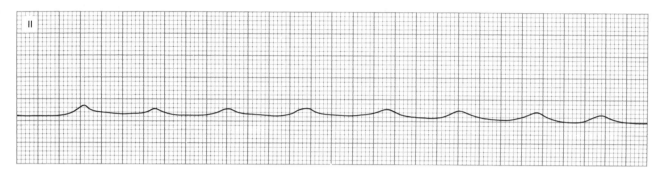

Code team members recognize the pattern as continued asystole. Mr. P. remains pulseless and unresponsive, so the team continues CPR.

A code team member should check the patient's pulse frequently during CPR, even with no ECG evidence of cardiac activity.

▼ Repeat epinephrine.

Five minutes have elapsed since the last dose, so the team leader administers another 1 mg of epinephrine.

Although epinephrine does not induce electrical or mechanical activity in asystole, it increases peripheral vascular resistance, aortic diastolic pressure, and coronary artery blood flow, which will benefit the patient if electrical and mechanical activity resume in the myocardium. The code team should repeat the dose every 5 minutes.

▼ Consider pacemaker therapy.

The code team leader decides to insert a ventricular pacemaker transvenously. After its insertion, Mr. P.'s rhythm is:

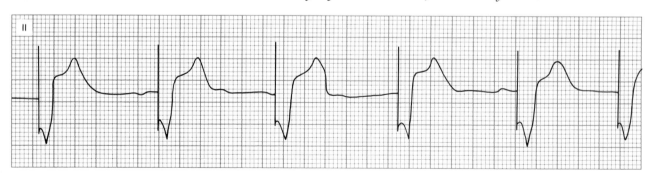

Team members recognize this pattern as a paced rhythm with a ventricular pacemaker. Mr. P.'s blood pressure is now 100/60 mm Hg. Although he remains unresponsive, a team member can

detect peripheral pulses. Mr. P. is transferred to the intensive care unit for post-resuscitation management, hemodynamic monitoring, and measurement of cardiac output.

Case study: Asystole resulting from ventricular fibrillation

Mrs. K., age 68, suddenly collapses while shopping with her daughter. Because Mrs. K. has a history of myocardial infarction and congestive heart failure, her daughter has learned basic life support techniques. She tells a store clerk to call the paramedics and, when she finds her mother pulseless and unresponsive, begins CPR. When the paramedics arrive, they place electrodes on Mrs. K.'s chest for cardiac monitoring.

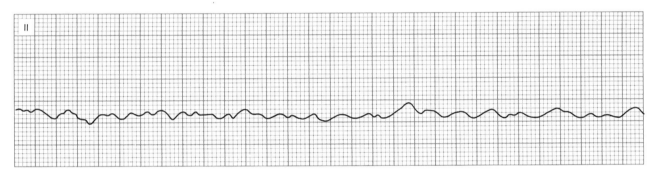

▼ Treat as ventricular fibrillation (see page 85).

The paramedics identify the rhythm as ventricular fibrillation. Mrs. K. remains pulseless, so the paramedics defibrillate her with 200 joules.

In an unwitnessed cardiac arrest, the appropriate intervention is to continue CPR until a defibrillator is available. At that time, defibrillation is appropriate. (See Chapter 7 for more information on ventricular fibrillation.)

After defibrillation, Mrs K. records the following rhythm on the monitor:

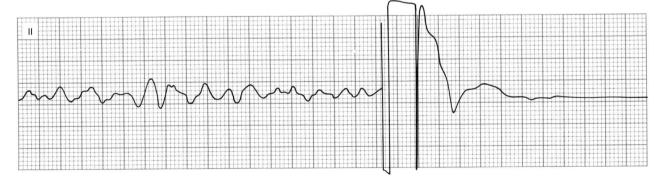

The paramedics identify the rhythm as asystole. Mrs. K. remains pulseless and unresponsive. The paramedics check the rhythm in another lead:

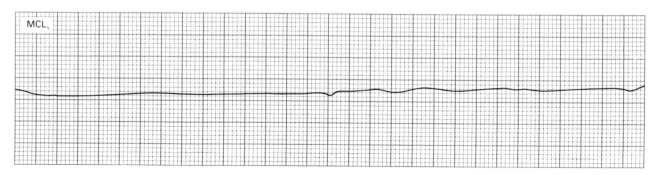

MCL₁

Continue CPR.

They identify the rhythm as asystole and continue CPR.

Defibrillating a patient with ventricular fibrillation can result in asystole. If the rhythm on the ECG monitor changes from ventricular fibrillation to asystole, code team members should:
• Check the patient for a pulse. Sometimes a loose lead can cause the flat line characteristic of asystole to appear on the monitor.
• Check the rhythm in another lead to confirm asystole. In some leads, fine ventricular fibrillation can look like asystole. Distinguishing between the two rhythms is important because defibrillation, the treatment of choice for ventricular fibrillation, is ineffective for asystole.

Establish I.V. line.
Administer epinephrine.

Asystole continues. Mrs. K. remains pulseless. The paramedics insert an 18G intracatheter into her right antecubital fossa and administer 0.5 mg of epinephrine by I.V. push.

If possible, a large-bore intracatheter should be inserted. Although an internal jugular or subclavian vein is preferred for drug administration, the antecubital vein is the first choice when starting an I.V. line during cardiac arrest, since inserting a jugular or subclavian line would interrupt CPR. Epinephrine is a first-line drug in managing cardiac arrest. It does not induce electrical or mechanical activity in the myocardium, but it does increase contractile strength, peripheral resistance, and coronary artery blood flow. Epinephrine exerts these effects through stimulation of alpha and beta receptors. (See Chapter 5 for a discussion of epinephrine's effects.)

Initiate endotracheal intubation.

En route to the hospital, the paramedics intubate Mrs. K. with a 7-mm endotracheal tube and ventilate her with a manual resuscitation bag and 100% O$_2$.

Intubation is an important step in resuscitation. Although ventilating the patient with a manual resuscitation bag can prevent severe hypoxemia, relying solely on this method is not recommended because endotracheal intubation promotes better oxygenation.

Despite the efforts of the paramedics, Mrs. K.'s rhythm continues:

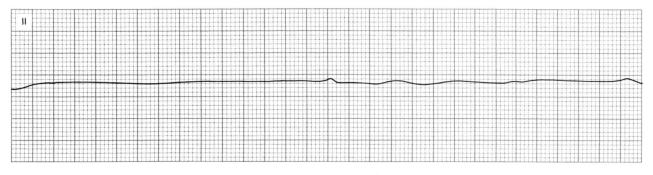

 Administer atropine.

On arrival in the emergency department (ED), Mrs. K. remains pulseless and unresponsive. CPR continues. The ED physician administers 1 mg of atropine by I.V. push and orders blood drawn for ABG analysis and electrolyte studies.

Atropine is administered at this point in an attempt to reverse severe parasympathetic stimulation of the heart. ABG values help assess oxygenation and acid-base status of the myocardium. Depending on the ABG results, sodium bicarbonate may be administered. Venous blood is drawn to determine whether an electrolyte imbalance contributed to the ventricular asystole.

 Repeat epinephrine.

The team repeats the epinephrine dose. ABG values for Mrs. K. are as follows: pH, 7.33; Pao_2, 130 mm Hg; $Paco_2$, 52 mm Hg; HCO_3, 21 mEq/liter. Electrolyte studies indicate the following: K^+, 3.8 (normally, 3.5 to 5.0); Na^+, 142 (normally, 136 to 145); Cl^-, 109 (normally, 98 to 106). Mrs. K's rhythm is:

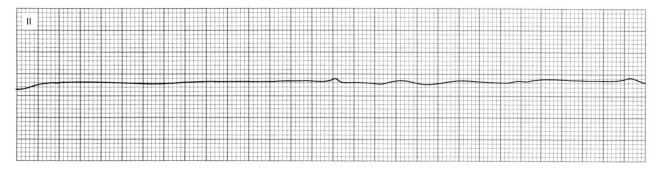

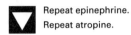

Repeat epinephrine.
Repeat atropine.

CPR continues. Mrs. K. remains pulseless and unresponsive. The epinephrine dose is repeated every 5 minutes, and another 1 mg of atropine is administered 5 minutes after the initial dose. The ECG monitor continues to show no sign of electrical activity. After several more minutes, the code is stopped and Mrs. K. is pronounced dead.

Although ventricular asystole usually is fatal, code team members must continue to support the patient's cardiac and respiratory function as long as the possibility exists that electrical and mechanical activity of the heart will return. The algorithm indicates that the code team should consider pacing the ventricle, an appropriate intervention if the ECG monitor shows occasional or intermittent electrical activity. In this case, the team ruled out pacing because they saw no indication that electrical activity would resume.

Case study: Asystole versus low-voltage ventricular fibrillation

Mr. L., age 47, comes into the ED complaining of chest pain. He has a 2-year history of angina pectoris, although his condition has been stable during this time, requiring one or two nitroglycerin tablets per month. In the last 2 weeks, however, he's needed two tablets per day. On admission to the ED, Mr. L. is given three nitroglycerin tablets, but his chest pain is unrelieved. A 12-lead ECG reveals ST segment elevation in the anterior leads. A nurse assesses his vital signs and records these results: blood pressure, 108/ 62 mm Hg; heart rate, 44 beats/minute; respiratory rate, 22 breaths/minute. Other staff members place electrodes on Mr. L. and attach the leads to the monitor, which shows the following rhythm:

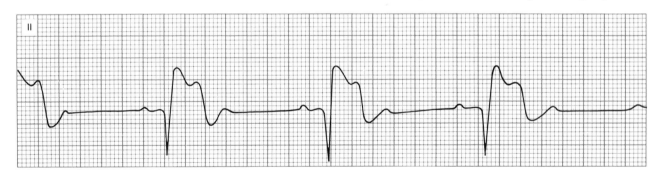

Identifying the rhythm as second-degree heart block with elevated ST segments, the ED physician instructs the nurse to start an I.V. line and administers 4 mg of morphine sulfate by I.V. push. As the nurse prepares to take Mr. L.'s blood pressure again, his eyes roll back and he becomes unconscious. The monitor now shows the following rhythm:

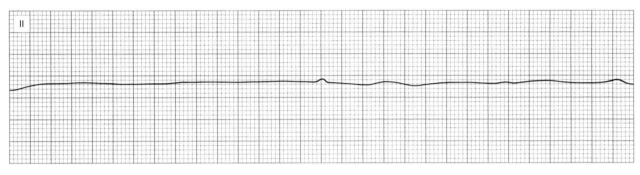

II

 Initiate CPR.

The physician identifies the rhythm as asystole. Mr. L. is pulseless and unresponsive, so the physician begins CPR while the nurse checks Mr. L.'s rhythm in another lead:

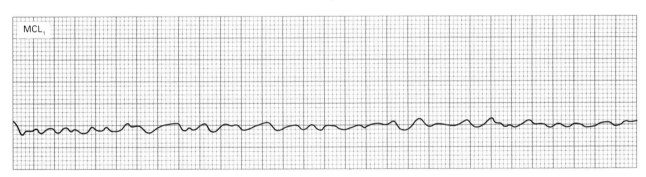

MCL₁

 Treat as ventricular fibrillation (see page 85).

The rhythm in this lead appears to be fine ventricular fibrillation. The physician charges the defibrillator and administers 200 joules to Mr. L.

Always check the rhythm in a second lead to confirm asystole because, as this case demonstrates, fine ventricular fibrillation can mimic asystole in some leads. Once rescuers confirm that the rhythm is ventricular fibrillation, their first priority is to defibrillate the patient. (See the algorithm on page 85 for further treatment of this rhythm.)

Study questions

Answers to study questions are on pages 126 and 127.

1. A neighbor finds Mr. D. lying on the sidewalk and calls for help. The paramedics place Mr. D. on a cardiac monitor and, en route to the hospital, report the rhythm as asystole. They are performing CPR when they bring him into the ED. What is your first intervention?

2. Mr. D. is placed on the cardiac monitor in the ED, which confirms asystole. The staff continues CPR. Describe the next two interventions.

3. Mr. D. remains pulseless and unresponsive. What are the next two interventions?

4. An ABG analysis of Mr. D. reveals the following: pH, 7.25; Pao_2, 88 mm Hg; $Paco_2$, 65 mm Hg; HCO_3, 20 mEq/liter. What should the staff do next?

5. If the staff decides to administer sodium bicarbonate, what would be the appropriate dose?

6. What is the next intervention?

7. You're caring for Mr. M., age 55, a patient who has recently undergone coronary artery bypass surgery, when he suddenly goes into ventricular fibrillation. Mr. M. is still on ventilatory support with 0.4 FIO_2 (40% O_2) at 12 breaths/minute. The code team arrives and defibrillates Mr. M. twice. The monitor displays the following rhythm:

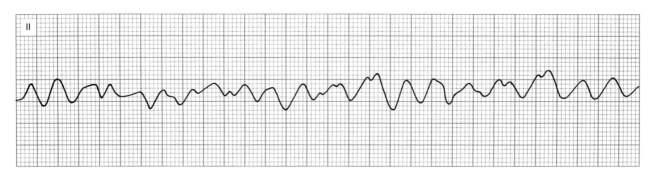

What are the next two interventions?

8. You check Mr. M.'s monitor and note the following rhythm:

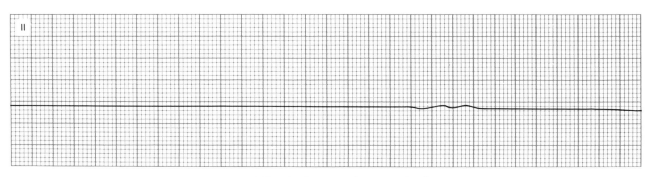

What is the next intervention?

9. The following rhythm appears on the monitor:

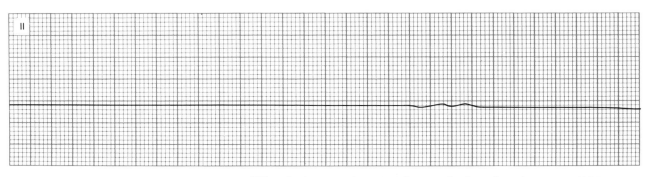

What is the next intervention, and what does it accomplish?

10. Since Mr. M. is already intubated, what would the next intervention be?

11. Describe two essential actions at this point in treating Mr. M.

12. Mr. M. continues in asystole. You draw some of his blood for laboratory analysis. Which laboratory tests are appropriate?

13. You check Mr. M.'s monitor and note the following rhythm:

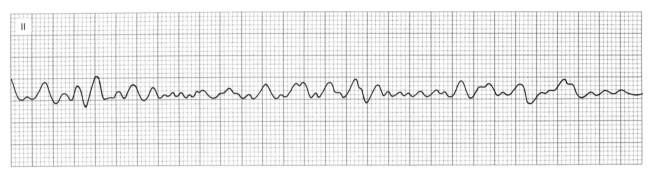

Interpret the rhythm, and describe the next appropriate intervention.

Answers to study questions

1. Check the patient's pulse.

2. Establish an I.V. line, and administer 0.5 to 1 mg of epinephrine by I.V. bolus.

3. Intubate the patient, and administer 1 mg of atropine by I.V. push.

4. Before considering sodium bicarbonate to correct the patient's acidosis, the staff should first ensure that the endotracheal tube is positioned correctly and that ventilations with the manual resuscitation bag are being administered properly. Increasing the rate and depth of ventilations usually improves oxygenation and corrects acidosis. Sodium bicarbonate should be administered only if the patient has severe metabolic acidosis.

5. 1 mEq/kg

6. Consider pacemaker insertion.

7. Check the patient's pulse. If the patient is pulseless, defibrillate.

8. Check the rhythm in another lead to confirm asystole.

9. Administer epinephrine, a first-line drug in managing cardiac arrest. Although epinephrine does not induce electrical or mechanical activity in the myocardium, it does increase contractile strength, peripheral vascular resistance, and coronary artery blood flow, which will benefit the patient if electrical and me-

chanical activity resume.

10. Administer 1 mg of atropine by I.V. push.

11. Continue CPR and check the patient's pulse.

12. ABG analysis is the most appropriate laboratory test, although venous blood could be drawn for electrolyte studies.

13. The rhythm is ventricular fibrillation. The next appropriate intervention would be to defibrillate the patient. Refer to the algorithm for ventricular fibrillation on page 85.

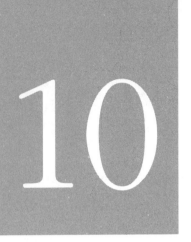

10

Electromechanical Dissociation

Electromechanical dissociation (EMD) refers to a condition in which the ECG shows cardiac electrical activity even though the patient shows no evidence of mechanical contraction. Primary EMD is associated with advanced cardiac disease or acute myocardial infarction. In secondary EMD, exsanguination, cardiac tamponade, or severe pulmonary embolism can result in an abrupt decrease in cardiac output. Prognosis is poor unless the underlying cause can be corrected.

The algorithm on the opposite page presents the established emergency treatment protocol for EMD. Case studies incorporating the algorithm's interventions follow.

ALGORITHM

ELECTROMECHANICAL DISSOCIATION

This algorithm presents the emergency measures to take for a patient with electromechanical dissociation (EMD). The steps are intended as guidelines, and some patients may require interventions not covered in these steps. The clinician should intubate the patient earlier than shown in this algorithm if it can be done simultaneously with other interventions. Keep in mind that sodium bicarbonate is not recommended for routine cardiac arrest.

Initiate cardiopulmonary resuscitation.

Establish an I.V. line.

Administer epinephrine (Adrenalin), 1:10,000, 0.5 to 1 mg by I.V. push.
(Repeat the dose every 5 minutes.)

▼

Insert endotracheal tube as soon as possible.

▼

Consider administering sodium bicarbonate.
(Repeat half of the original dose every 10 minutes.)

Consider these conditions as possible causes:
hypovolemia, cardiac tamponade, tension pneumothorax, hypoxemia, acidosis, and
pulmonary embolism.

Case study: EMD with hypovolemia

Mrs. M., age 85, is found in bed by her son and daughter-in-law, who went to her home when she repeatedly failed to answer their telephone calls. Although she is conscious, Mrs. M. appears weak and in need of medical attention, so her son calls 911. Paramedics arrive to find Mrs. M. responsive to touch. Her pulse is rapid and weak; her blood pressure, 80/54 mm Hg. The paramedics place electrodes on her chest and connect her to an ECG monitor, which shows the following rhythm:

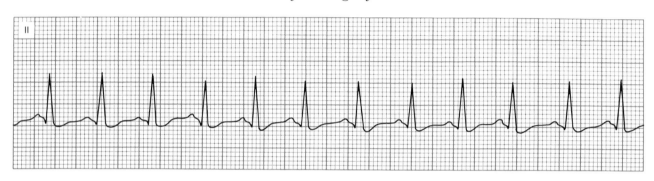

The paramedics identify the rhythm as sinus tachycardia and prepare to transport Mrs. M. to the emergency department (ED). En route, she suddenly gasps and loses consciousness. The monitor now shows this rhythm:

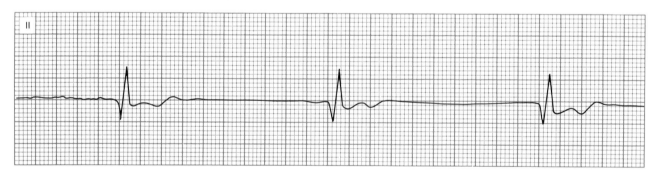

 Initiate CPR.

The paramedics recognize this as an idioventricular rhythm, but Mrs. M. has no pulse. Suspecting EMD, the paramedics begin cardiopulmonary resuscitation (CPR).

In EMD, mechanical contraction is absent and the patient lacks effective cardiac output, even though the ECG shows evidence of electrical activity. This electrical activity may be organized or irregular. In either case, basic life support techniques must be instituted.

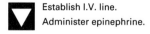 Establish I.V. line.
Administer epinephrine.

The paramedics start an I.V. line and administer 0.5 mg of epinephrine (Adrenalin) 1:10,000 by I.V. push.

Establishing an I.V. line enables rescuers to administer drugs and fluids during a cardiac emergency. Epinephrine, the drug of choice for EMD, increases systemic vascular resistance and heart rate, elevates arterial blood pressure, strengthens myocardial contractility and automaticity, and improves coronary artery blood flow. The recommended dose is 0.5 to 1 mg, depending on the patient's condition and body size. (See Chapter 5, Pharmacologic Therapy, for more detailed information on epinephrine.)

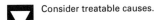 Initiate intubation.

Mrs. M.'s rhythm remains idioventricular, and she still has no palpable pulse when she arrives at the hospital. The ED staff physician intubates Mrs. M. with an endotracheal tube.

Although a manual resuscitation bag can prevent severe hypoxemia, endotracheal intubation should be instituted as soon as possible to ensure adequate ventilation and prevent acid-base abnormalities.

Consider treatable causes.

ED staff members continue CPR efforts on Mrs. M., who remains pulseless. The physician inserts a central I.V. line into the jugular vein for drug administration, noting that Mrs. M.'s neck veins are flat and that a brisk back flow of blood from the jugular vein does not occur. Next, the physician orders blood drawn for arterial blood gas (ABG) analysis. A nurse then auscultates Mrs. M.'s lung sounds.

Successful treatment of EMD depends on supporting the patient's ventilation and circulation while trying to find a treatable cause of EMD. In a patient with adequate fluid volume (normovolemia), venous pressure typically increases during CPR; thus, back flow of blood from the jugular vein would be expected when an I.V. line is inserted. Absence of this back flow suggests hypovolemia, one of the treatable conditions associated with secondary EMD. ABG analysis helps assess the patient's oxygenation and detect acid-base imbalances (to correct severe imbalances, the physician may consider administering sodium bicarbonate). By auscultating lung sounds, the nurse can ensure accurate placement of the endotracheal tube and detect evidence of pneumothorax (such as absent lung sounds on one side of the chest), another condition associated with EMD.

Staff members continue CPR. Mrs. M.'s lung sounds show no evidence of pneumothorax. ABG analysis yields these results: pH, 7.33; Po_2, 110 mm Hg; Pco_2, 50 mm Hg; HCO_3, 19 mEq/liter. The physician instructs the nurse to administer 1,000 ml of lactated Ringer's solution I.V.

A Pco_2 of 50 mm Hg indicates mild metabolic and respiratory acidosis, which can be corrected by increasing the rate and depth of ventilations. Because the patient's oxygenation is adequate and pneumothorax has been ruled out, I.V. fluid is administered to test another possibility—if ventricular filling and subsequent stroke volume increase in response to I.V. fluid administration, hypovolemia is the likely cause of EMD.

 Repeat epinephrine.

The physician asks the nurse to administer 1 mg of epinephrine I.V.

As noted in the algorithm for EMD, rescuers should repeat the epinephrine dose every 5 minutes. Research suggests that a higher dose (5 mg) of epinephrine may be needed to produce the most beneficial effects, although the higher dose is not currently part of the algorithm.

Staff members discontinue CPR efforts momentarily to assess Mrs. M.'s condition. Her pulse is weak. She has a palpated blood pressure of 90 mm Hg.

Blood pressure is difficult to auscultate when a patient has a weak pulse. Use the following method to palpate the blood pressure:
• Palpate the brachial pulse.
• Inflate the blood pressure cuff until the pulse is no longer palpable.
• Slowly deflate the cuff.
• Note the manometer reading at the point when the pulse is palpated. This is the "palpated blood pressure."

The ECG monitor shows the following rhythm:

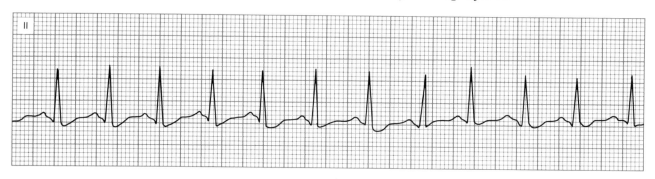

The physician identifies the rhythm as sinus tachycardia and instructs the nurse to administer another 1,000 ml of lactated Ringer's solution. Other ED staff members prepare to transfer Mrs. M. to the intensive care unit (ICU).

The initial infusion of lactated Ringer's solution probably increased the patient's ventricular filling time and stroke volume, but because her pulse remained thready, the physician prescribed additional fluid. Since the patient has not regained consciousness, she will be placed on a mechanical ventilator in the ICU until her condition stabilizes. Additionally, a team member will insert a pulmonary artery line to monitor her fluid status.

Case study: EMD with pneumothorax

 Initiate CPR.

While surfing with friends, Mr. S. is struck in the head by his surfboard, which knocks him unconscious. After his friends bring him ashore, one of them, a lifeguard, determines that Mr. S. is pulseless. He immediately begins CPR and continues his efforts as the friends drive Mr. S. to a hospital several miles away. CPR is in progress when Mr. S. is admitted to the ED. Team members institute cardiac monitoring and observe the following rhythm:

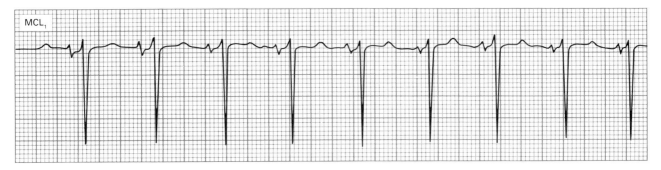

MCL₁

An ED nurse identifies this as a normal sinus rhythm, although Mr. S. remains pulseless, with no evidence of cardiac contraction. The team leader diagnoses the condition as EMD.

Electrical activity on the monitor without corresponding evidence of cardiac mechanical contraction in the patient supports the diagnosis. This situation illustrates the importance of checking for a pulse even when the cardiac monitor shows apparently normal electrical activity.

 Establish an I.V. line.

The team leader directs members to continue CPR and to start an I.V. line.

CPR must be continued to support the patient's ventilation and circulation during EMD. Establishing an I.V. line enables rescuers to administer medications and fluids.

 Administer epinephrine.

The team leader asks a nurse to administer 0.5 mg of epinephrine 1:10,000 by I.V. push.

Among its many beneficial effects, epinephrine promotes peripheral vasoconstriction, improves coronary blood flow, strengthens myocardial contractility, and increases automaticity.

 Initiate intubation.
Consider treatable causes.

The team leader institutes endotracheal intubation and orders a chest X-ray for Mr. S.

Intubating the patient as quickly as possible improves ventilation and helps prevent acidosis. The chest X-ray not only confirms proper endotracheal tube placement but also can help the team determine a treatable cause of EMD. The most common treatable conditions associated with EMD are tension pneumothorax, cardiac tamponade, and hypovolemia.

On the monitor, the nurse views this rhythm:

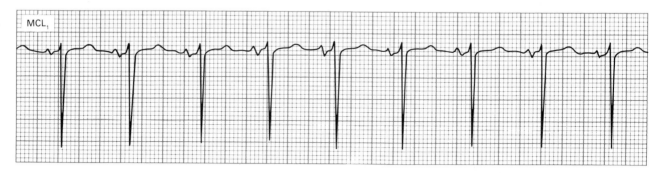

▼ Repeat epinephrine.

The monitor continues to show sinus rhythm, even though Mr. S. remains pulseless. His chest X-ray shows a left pneumothorax with moderate tracheal shift. The team leader performs a needle aspiration, inserts a chest tube, and administers another 0.5 mg of epinephrine.

Tension pneumothorax is treated with a needle aspiration to relieve the pressure that builds up within the pleural space. Chest tube insertion assists with reexpansion of the lung. As noted in the algorithm, the epinephrine dose should be repeated every 5 minutes.

After the second dose of epinephrine, the following rhythm appears on the monitor:

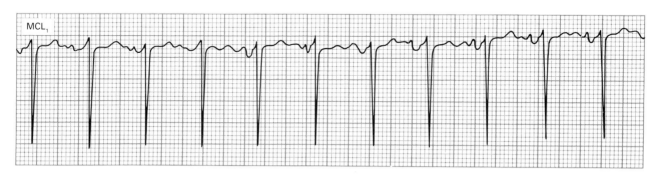

The team leader identifies the rhythm as sinus tachycardia. Mr. S., although still unconscious, now has a pulse. His blood pressure is 92/66 mm Hg. Team members transfer Mr. S. to the ICU for further observation and treatment.

Case study: EMD with cardiac tamponade

Mr. D., who underwent coronary artery bypass graft surgery yesterday, is recuperating in the hospital's cardiopulmonary unit. He is still intubated and has a pulmonary artery catheter in place. A nurse checking his progress observes this rhythm on the cardiac monitor:

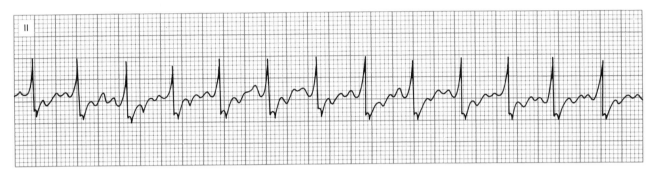

The nurse identifies the rhythm as sinus tachycardia. She is concerned because Mr. D.'s heart sounds are distant, his cardiac output has diminished considerably from the last few measurements, and venous pressure is elevated. After paging the physician to alert him to Mr. D.'s status, she observes the following rhythm on the monitor:

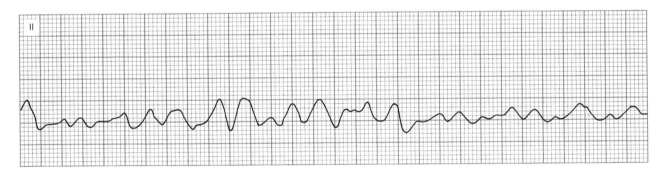

 No pulse. Treat as ventricular fibrillation (see page 85).
Defibrillate with 200 joules.

Identifying the rhythm as ventricular fibrillation (VF), the nurse assesses Mr. D. but cannot detect a pulse. She shakes him and calls out his name, but he does not respond. The physician, who arrived moments earlier, immediately defibrillates Mr. D. with 200 joules.

Defibrillation is the definitive treatment for VF. Note that rescuers must check for a pulse before defibrillating a patient. (See Chapter 6, Electrical and Mechanical Interventions, and Chapter 7, Ventricular Fibrillation, for more information.)

After the first defibrillation, this rhythm appears on the monitor:

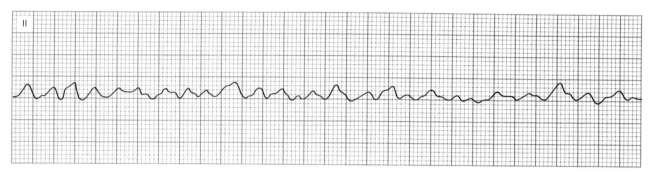

▼ Check pulse.
Defibrillate with 200 to 300 joules.

VF continues, so the physician defibrillates Mr. D. again, this time increasing the energy level to 300 joules.

If VF continues after the first defibrillation, the standard protocol is to defibrillate the patient again, using 200 to 300 joules. The chances for success increase with successive defibrillations because each attempt further decreases transthoracic resistance.

By now, other staff members have arrived to help. The team observes the following rhythm on the monitor:

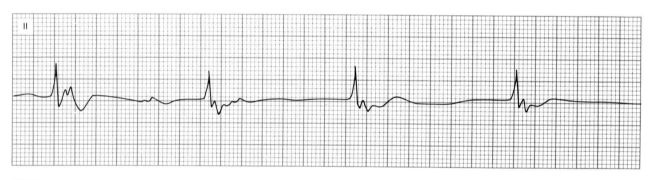

▼ No pulse. Treat as EMD.
Initiate CPR.
Administer epinephrine.

The ECG monitor shows a junctional rhythm, but the nurse cannot detect a pulse in Mr. D. Diagnosing the condition as EMD, the physician instructs staff members to begin CPR and administers 1 mg of epinephrine by I.V. push.

As noted earlier, when electrical activity appears on the monitor even though the patient has no pulse, EMD is the appropriate diagnosis. As soon as rescuers determine that the patient's heart is not contracting, they must initiate basic life support measures. The physician administers epinephrine to increase systemic vascular resistance and stimulate cardiac contraction.

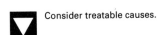
Consider treatable causes.

Despite the team's efforts, Mr. D.'s pulse does not return. The physician decides to perform pericardiocentesis.

Whenever EMD occurs, the team must find and treat the underlying cause. Otherwise, the patient's chances of recovery are poor. Distant heart sounds, diminished cardiac output, and elevated venous pressure suggest that the patient has cardiac tamponade, a condition that can develop after cardiac surgery. Other conditions associated with EMD include hypovolemia, tension pneumothorax, hypoxemia, acidosis, and pulmonary embolism.

Carefully inserting the needle, the physician removes 200 ml of fluid from the pericardial space. On the ECG monitor, the team now observes the following rhythm:

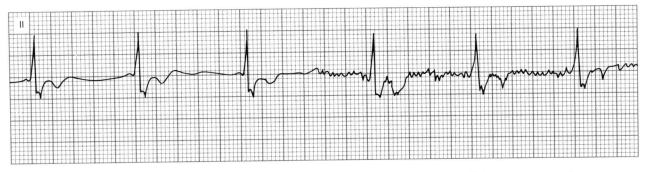

Mr. D. has a normal sinus rhythm, and the nurse can detect a weak pulse. Blood pressure is 112/80 mm Hg; cardiac index, 3.0. The physician decides to take Mr. D. back to surgery to determine and correct the cause of bleeding.

Study questions

Answers to study questions are on pages 140 and 141.

1. Team members are caring for Mrs. J. in the critical care unit (CCU) after she has had an anterior wall myocardial infarction. The team is inserting a pulmonary artery line when the following rhythm appears on the monitor:

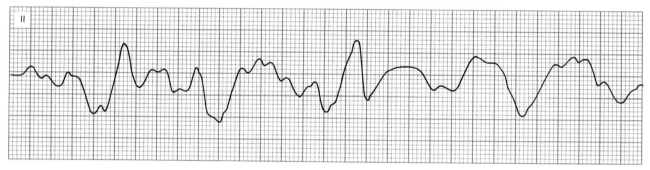

The team leader identifies the rhythm as VF. Name the first two measures the team should take for this life-threatening emergency.

2. Mrs. J. has no pulse, so the team leader directs other members to prepare for defibrillation. After the first attempt, team members observe the following rhythm:

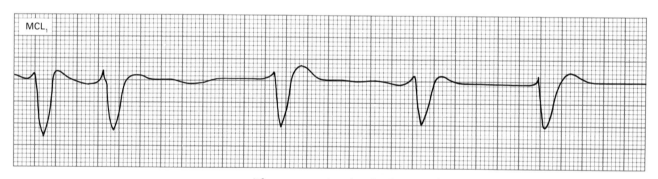

They recognize the rhythm as idioventricular. What should the team do next?

3. Mrs. J. remains pulseless and unresponsive, and her rhythm does not change. How would you assess her condition?

4. Name the possible causes of this patient's condition.

5. What is the next appropriate intervention?

6. Describe the next two interventions the team should carry out.

7. On the ECG monitor, the team now observes this rhythm:

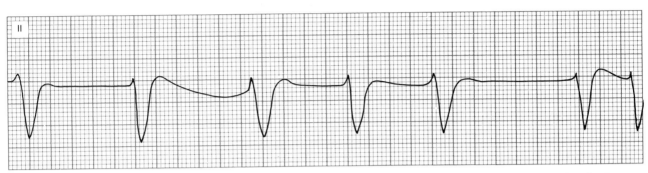

The team leader identifies it as an accelerated ventricular rhythm. What should the team do next?

8. Mrs. J. remains pulseless and unresponsive. Name the next appropriate intervention.

9. What is the prognosis for Mrs. J.'s condition?

10. Discuss additional interventions that the team should consider.

11. Friends of Mrs. R. bring her to the ED after she falls from a ladder while painting her house. ED staff members place electrodes on Mrs. R. and connect her to an ECG monitor, which displays the following rhythm:

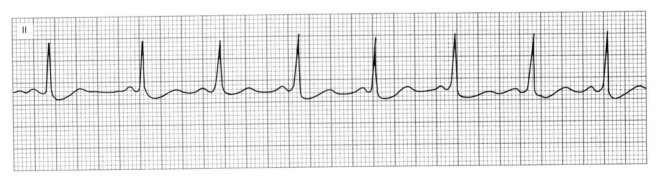

Interpret the rhythm.

12. Discuss important assessments the ED staff should make in caring for Mrs. R.

13. While staff members are assessing Mrs. R.'s condition, she begins

to gasp and then loses consciousness. The ECG monitor shows the following rhythm:

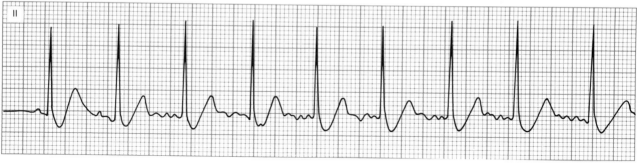

Staff members recognize this as sinus rhythm. State the next appropriate intervention.

14. Mrs. R. has no pulse. Discuss the next several steps that the ED staff should take if her condition does not change.

15. Mrs. R.'s clinical status remains unchanged, and the ED staff must quickly find and correct the cause of EMD. Given the nature of her injuries, discuss the causes that the ED staff will probably consider.

Answers to study questions

1. When VF occurs, rescuers should first check the patient for a pulse. If a pulse cannot be detected, the next step is to defibrillate the patient with 200 joules.

2. Recheck the patient's pulse.

3. Electrical activity on the ECG monitor (indicated by the idioventricular rhythm) without corresponding evidence of mechanical contraction (the patient is pulseless) supports a diagnosis of EMD.

4. Hypovolemia, cardiac tamponade (from ventricular rupture), hypoxemia, acidosis, or pulmonary embolism may have caused the EMD. Tension pneumothorax can also cause EMD, although the facts presented in the study question do not support tension pneumothorax as a probable cause in this case.

5. Begin CPR.

6. Establish an I.V. line (if not done earlier), and administer 0.5 to 1 mg of epinephrine by I.V. push.

7. Recheck the patient to determine whether a pulse has returned, and continue CPR, regularly assessing whether basic life support efforts are being performed correctly. These two steps cannot be overemphasized.

8. Initiate endotracheal intubation.

9. The prognosis for EMD is poor unless its cause can be found and corrected.

10. The team leader may decide to draw blood for ABG analysis (which can detect acidosis, inadequate oxygenation, and pulmonary embolism) and order a chest X-ray (to determine placement of an endotracheal tube and pulmonary artery line). While continuing basic life support measures to support the patient's ventilation and circulation, the team should also consider hypovolemia and ventricular rupture as possible causes of the EMD.

11. The monitor shows a normal sinus rhythm.

12. The staff should perform cardiovascular (pulse, heart sounds, and peripheral circulation), pulmonary (lung sounds and possible chest trauma), and neurologic (possible head injury) assessments.

13. Check the patient's pulse.

14. Because the ECG monitor continues to show a normal sinus rhythm even after ED staff members have determined that the patient has no pulse, EMD is the probable diagnosis. Therefore, until the staff can find and correct the cause of EMD, they should initiate and maintain CPR, establish an I.V. line, administer 0.5 to 1 mg of epinephrine 1:10,000 by I.V. push, institute endotracheal intubation, and regularly check the patient's pulse.

15. Given the nature of the patient's injuries, the ED staff should consider the treatable conditions associated with EMD—hypoxemia, acidosis, hypovolemia (from blood loss), cardiac tamponade (from cardiac trauma), and tension pneumothorax (from broken ribs). Massive pulmonary embolism can also cause EMD, but traumatic causes are more likely in this case.

11

Paroxysmal Supraventricular Tachycardia and Atrial Arrhythmias

Paroxysmal supraventricular tachycardia (PSVT)

develops when a reentry circuit involving the atria, the

AV junction, or an accessory pathway is established.

Treatment consists of vagal maneuvers, drug therapy,

cardioversion, or cardiac pacing. Atrial fibrillation,

atrial flutter with varying conduction, and multifocal

atrial tachycardia warrant similar treatment.

The algorithm on the opposite page presents the

established emergency treatment protocol for PSVT.

Case studies incorporating the algorithm's interven-

tions follow.

PAROXYSMAL SUPRAVENTRICULAR TACHYCARDIA

This algorithm presents the emergency measures to take for a patient with paroxysmal supraventricular tachycardia (PSVT). If PSVT recurs after conversion to a normal rhythm, the clinician should not repeat cardioversion attempts but may order sedatives if time and the patient's condition permit. A stable patient is one who maintains adequate cardiac output, as evidenced by a systolic blood pressure above 90 mm Hg, palpable pulses, and a normal mental status. An unstable patient may present with shock or congestive heart failure, lose consciousness, or show other signs of inadequate peripheral perfusion. Atrial fibrillation with a rapid ventricular response or atrial flutter may cause similar signs of inadequate cardiac output. Although these rhythms do not meet the criteria for PSVT, rescuers may use antiarrhythmic drug therapy or cardioversion at lower energy levels (25 to 75 joules).

For an unstable patient

Perform synchronized cardioversion at 75 to 100 joules.
▼
Repeat cardioversion at 200 joules.
▼
Repeat cardioversion at 360 joules.
▼
Correct underlying abnormalities.
▼
Combine pharmacologic therapy with cardioversion.

For a stable patient

Perform vagal maneuvers, such as Valsalva's maneuver or carotid sinus massage.
▼
Administer 5 mg of verapamil (Calan) I.V. (Double the dose in 15 to 20 minutes.)
▼
Perform cardioversion, administer digoxin (Lanoxin) or beta blockers, or institute cardiac pacing as indicated.

Case study: Stable PSVT

Mrs. W., age 36, comes to the emergency department (ED) after experiencing a sudden onset of palpitations at her secretarial job. On admission, she appears anxious and complains of dizziness, but the problem seems to subside once she is placed on the gurney. Trim and muscular, Mrs. W. tells the admissions nurse that she has no history of cardiovascular problems, proudly stating that she exercises regularly.

The nurse connects Mrs. W. to an electrocardiogram (ECG) monitor and records her vital signs: blood pressure, 100/60 mm Hg; heart rate, 150 beats/minute and regular; respiratory rate, 22 breaths/minute, with lungs clear on auscultation. The monitor shows the following rhythm:

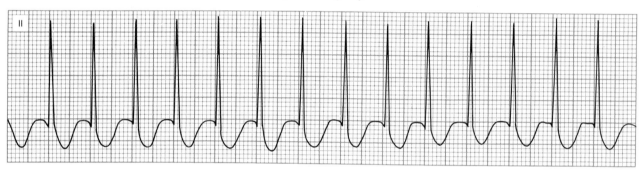

The nurse cannot see clear P waves in the rhythm and accurately interprets it as supraventricular tachycardia, or, more precisely, PSVT, based on the sudden onset of palpitations. She notifies the ED physician, who has arrived to examine Mrs. W.

More than one atrial impulse may be associated with each QRS complex because, as the rate becomes faster, P waves may merge with QRS complexes and T waves. The ventricular rate of 150 beats/minute is also characteristic of atrial flutter with a 2:1 conduction.

▼ Perform vagal maneuvers.

The nurse administers oxygen at 5 liters/minute by nasal cannula. The physician then instructs Mrs. W. to bear down and perform Valsalva's maneuver, but this has no effect on the rhythm. He then performs carotid sinus massage (CSM).

Valsalva's maneuver and CSM are appropriate initial interventions in treating PSVT if the patient is hemodynamically stable. By increasing vagal tone, these maneuvers may convert the arrhythmia to a normal sinus rhythm or create a block in the AV node to slow the patient's ventricular rate. The slower ventricular response may enable the ED staff to visualize blocked P waves.

The CSM performed by the physician triggers this change in Mrs. W.'s rhythm:

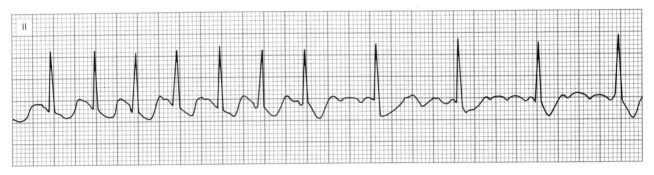

Identifying the rhythm as atrial flutter with a 4:1 conduction ratio, the nurse increases the gain on the ECG monitor, which now shows the following:

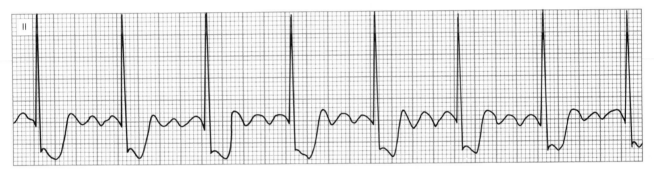

Atrial flutter continues, only more apparent now because the flutter waves are easily visualized. The nurse rechecks Mrs. W.'s blood pressure (120/70 mm Hg) and heart rate (75 beats/minute).

CSM can trigger a block in the AV node, thereby slowing the ventricular rate. Because atrial flutter causes loss of effective atrial contraction, the slower ventricular rate allows more time for passive ventricular filling and usually results in increased cardiac output.

After 8 minutes, Mrs. W.'s original rhythm—PSVT with a 2:1 atrial conduction—returns. The physician decides to initiate drug therapy, administering 5 mg of verapamil (Calan) I.V.

▼ Administer verapamil.

Verapamil, a calcium channel blocker, slows the influx of calcium into the cell, thus slowing conduction of electrical impulses through the AV node and lengthening the refractory period.

Within 10 minutes, Mrs. W.'s rhythm converts to the following:

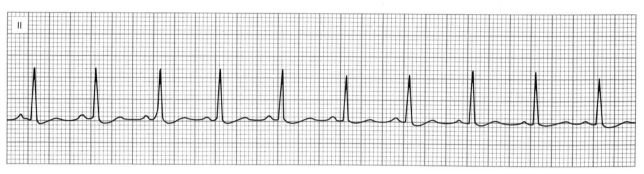

A normal sinus rhythm returns. The nurse rechecks Mrs. W.'s blood pressure (124/76 mm Hg) and heart rate (98 beats/minute). The physician orders additional antiarrhythmic therapy to prevent a recurrence.

Case study: Unstable SVT

Miss P., a 58-year-old accountant, is transported to the ED by paramedics responding to her co-worker's 911 call. At the office, Miss P. had been complaining of chest pressure and felt as if she were going to pass out. Now, she appears pale; her skin is cool and moist.

Responding to a nurse's questions, Miss P. states that she weighs 150 lb (68 kg) and has recently felt unusually stressed on the job. She continues to feel light-headed. ED staff members administer oxygen at 5 liters/minute via nasal cannula and infuse an I.V. solution of dextrose 5% in water at a keep-vein-open rate. Miss P. has been transported with an ECG monitor, which shows the following rhythm:

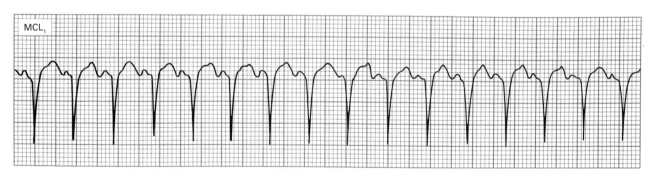

The staff identify the rhythm as supraventricular tachycardia (SVT), possibly an atrial tachycardia because P waves seem to be visible. A nurse checks Miss P.'s vital signs: blood pressure, 90/58 mm Hg; heart rate, 180 beats/minute and regular; respiratory rate, 24 breaths/minute, with normal breath sounds. The ED physician performs CSM, with no change in the rhythm. Miss P. again feels that she is going to pass out. Her blood pressure drops to 86/50 mm Hg. The physician decides to treat the condition as unstable SVT and instructs the staff to prepare Miss P. for cardioversion.

In unstable PSVT or SVT, rescuers should attempt to convert the arrhythmia as soon as possible. In this case, the patient's symptoms (hypotension and light-headedness) suggest inadequate cardiac output and thus warrant cardioversion (synchronized countershock), which can convert the arrhythmia more rapidly than pharmacologic therapy.

▼ Perform cardioversion at 75 to 100 joules.

The physician orders 10 mg of diazepam (Valium) I.V. and explains the procedure to Miss P., who continues to feel light-headed. Other staff members ensure that the I.V. line is patent before administering the diazepam. The physician then performs cardioversion at 100 joules:

MCL₁

The synchronized countershock converts the SVT to a sinus rhythm.

Cardioversion uses a synchronized countershock to deliver electrical energy on the QRS complex. This prevents delivery of the countershock on the T wave, which could worsen the arrhythmia.

The nurse rechecks Miss P.'s blood pressure (106/68 mm Hg) and heart rate (110 beats/minute). Although drowsy from the diazepam, Miss P. responds to verbal stimuli. During the next 10 minutes, the nurse begins to note frequent premature atrial complexes (PACs) along with sinus tachycardia:

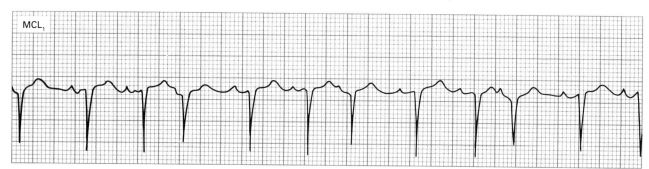

▼ Initiate pharmacologic therapy.

Because Miss P. arouses easily and can swallow, the physician decides to start her on oral quinidine (Quinidex) therapy and administers 200 mg as an initial dose.

After SVT converts to a sinus rhythm, a physician may initiate antiarrhythmic therapy to prevent a recurrence and additionally may order a 12-lead ECG, which can help detect a preexcitation syndrome, determine the cause of SVT, or indicate its most effective treatment.

Case study: Atrial fibrillation

Mr. T., a 68-year-old retired firefighter, is admitted to the critical care unit (CCU) with congestive heart failure. A nurse records his weight (176 lb [80 kg]) and vital signs (blood pressure, 120/90 mm Hg; heart rate, 180 beats/minute; respiratory rate, 36 breaths/ minute, with rales at the lung bases). Sitting in a high Fowler's position, he appears dyspneic. While oxygen is administered via nasal cannula at 4 liters/minute, he is connected to an ECG monitor, which shows the following rhythm:

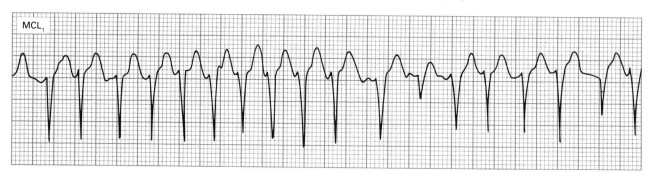

The nurse recognizes the rapid, irregular rhythm characteristic of uncontrolled atrial fibrillation and alerts the physician to Mr. T.'s clinical status.

Atrial fibrillation can either cause or result from pump failure, a condition with which the arrhythmia is commonly associated. Ventricular failure increases pressure within the atria, stretching and irritating the atrial wall and causing atrial ectopy.

The physician orders 0.5 mg of digoxin (Lanoxin) I.V. and, after 20 minutes pass with no change in the rhythm, orders 40 mg of furosemide (Lasix) I.V. The nurse inserts an indwelling urinary catheter, then rechecks Mr. T.'s blood pressure (104/80 mm Hg) and respiratory rate (40 breaths/minute, with increased congestion).

The physician administers digoxin in this case because the patient has congestive heart failure. Digoxin not only slows conduction at the AV node but also improves myocardial contractility, although its therapeutic benefits do not fully take effect for several hours. Furosemide is administered to induce diuresis, which would decrease the patient's pulmonary congestion and dyspnea. The indwelling catheter monitors the patient's urine output.

Considering Mr. T.'s lowered blood pressure and elevated respiratory rate, the physician instructs CCU staff members to prepare for cardioversion, explains the procedure to Mr. T., and then administers 5 mg of diazepam I.V. for sedation.

Cardioversion is the appropriate intervention to convert atrial fibrillation in an unstable patient. The digoxin administered earlier will help maintain a normal rhythm after conversion. Note, however, that cardioversion is not the treatment of choice when digoxin toxicity is suspected in a patient already taking the drug. Digoxin toxicity increases the risk that asystole or a ventricular arrhythmia will occur in response to countershock.

▼ Prepare to initiate cardioversion at 75 to 100 joules.

The physician activates the synchronizer switch on the defibrillator and sets the energy level for 75 joules. Before the team's first attempt at cardioversion, however, Mr. T.'s rhythm suddenly changes:

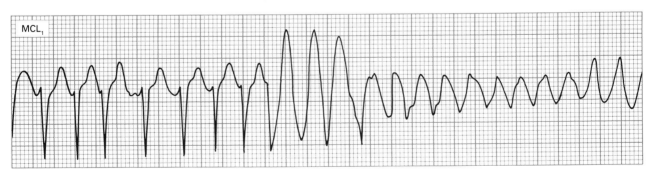

MCL₁

Treat pulseless VT as ventricular fibrillation (see page 85).
Defibrillate with 200 joules.

Staff members observe a short burst of ventricular tachycardia, followed by torsades de pointes. The nurse announces that she cannot detect a pulse in Mr. T. The physician turns off the synchronizer switch, increases the energy setting to 200 joules, instructs the staff to stand clear, applies the defibrillator paddles, and depresses the buttons:

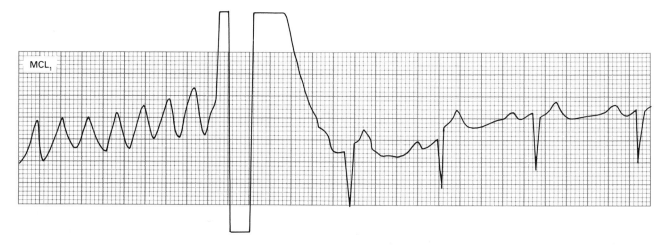

MCL₁

Mr. T. converts to sinus rhythm with a first-degree AV block. The PR interval is 0.24 second. His blood pressure is 90/60 mm Hg; heart rate, 72 beats/minute; respiratory rate, 22 breaths/minute. Within 5 minutes, his heart rate rises to 80 beats/minute. His sinus rhythm now has frequent PACs:

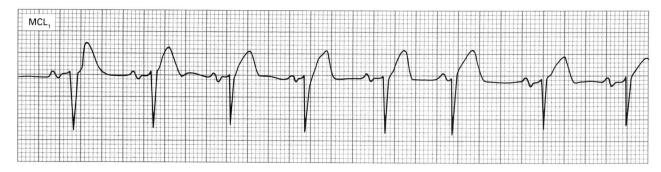

MCL₁

Mr. T. is alert and responsive. The indwelling catheter has drained 400 ml of urine, indicating diuresis. The physician orders 400 mg of procainamide (Procan) I.V., to be infused at a slow rate of 20 mg/minute.

Procainamide is an appropriate antiarrhythmic agent for this patient because it effectively treats both ventricular and supraventricular ectopy.

Study questions

Answers to study questions are on page 153.

1. Mrs. L., age 45, walks into the ED, seeking treatment for palpitations and dizziness. A nurse records the woman's weight (130 lb [59 kg]) and vital signs (blood pressure, 100/60 mm Hg; heart rate, 166 beats/minute and regular; respiratory rate, 28 breaths/minute, with lungs clear on auscultation). Mrs. L. tells the nurse that she has no history of cardiovascular problems and has never been connected to an ECG before. On the monitor, the following rhythm appears:

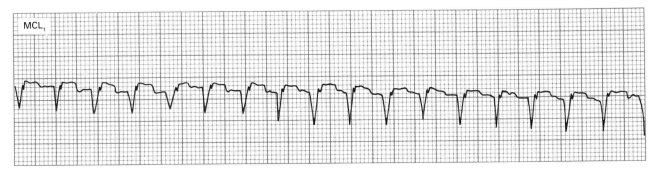

Interpret the rhythm.

2. Name two initial interventions that would be appropriate for Mrs. L.'s condition.

3. The ED physician performs CSM, which changes the rhythm to the one shown here:

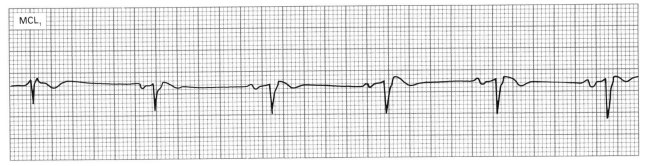

Interpret the rhythm.

4. If vagal maneuvers do not effectively convert stable PSVT, discuss the next therapeutic intervention that a physician might consider.

5. Mr. K., age 62, is admitted to the CCU after suffering an inferior wall myocardial infarction. The ECG monitor has shown a sinus rhythm for the past few hours, but now his rhythm suddenly changes:

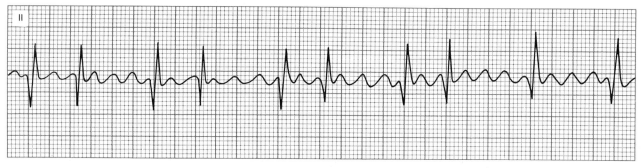

Interpret the rhythm.

6. The nurse administers oxygen at 6 liters/minute via nasal cannula and records Mr. K.'s blood pressure (110/84 mm Hg) and heart rate (100 beats/minute and irregular). Respiratory assessment reveals rales at both lung bases. The nurse notifies the physician of Mr. K.'s status. Identify two therapeutic interventions that should be considered.

7. Why must the staff convert Mr. K.'s arrhythmia to a normal rhythm as quickly as possible?

8. Is 4:1 conduction of atria flutter more desirable than 2:1 conduction? Justify your answer.

Answers to study questions

1. Supraventricular tachycardia

2. Administer oxygen, and perform vagal maneuvers (such as Valsalva's maneuver and CSM).

3. Sinus bradycardia

4. Initiate pharmacologic therapy with verapamil, digoxin, or beta blockers, such as propranolol (Inderal).

5. Atrial flutter with 2:1 and 4:1 conduction

6. Administer 0.25 to 0.5 mg of digoxin I.V., or perform cardioversion.

7. Atrial flutter results in a loss of atrial-ventricular synchrony, or atrial kick, which reduces cardiac output. Additionally, mural emboli may form within the atria. Atrial flutter commonly degenerates to atrial fibrillation.

8. Yes. With 4:1 conduction of atrial flutter, the ventricular rate is likely to fall within a normal range, typically 70 to 80 beats/minute. A 2:1 conduction, on the other hand, usually produces rates of about 150 beats/minute. The slower rate produced by 4:1 conduction requires less oxygen consumption and is more beneficial to the patient's hemodynamic status.

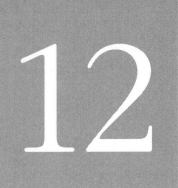

12

Bradycardia and Atrioventricular Blocks

A slow heart rate can be caused by various conditions, ranging from normal slowing of the firing rate of the SA node, to ischemia or drug depression of the SA or AV node. The clinician must identify the rhythm in-volved—sinus bradycardia, junctional escape rhythm, or second- or third-degree AV block—and then assess the patient's hemodynamic status to de-termine appropriate interventions.

The algorithm on the opposite page presents the established emergency treatment protocol for brady-cardia. Case studies incorporating the algorithm's interventions follow.

BRADYCARDIA

This algorithm presents the emergency measures to take for a patient with bradycardia (heart rate less than 60 beats/minute). Some patients may require additional interventions not covered in these steps. Before attempting the interventions below, the clinician could deliver a single chest thump or encourage the patient to cough; either may stimulate sufficient electrical activity to improve cardiac output. Signs and symptoms in the algorithm refer to hypotension, premature ventricular complexes, altered mental status, chest pain, dyspnea, and ischemia. The clinician uses an external pacemaker and isoproterenol (Isuprel) administration as temporary measures until a transvenous pacemaker is inserted.

Determine the cause of bradycardia.

▼

If the patient has sinus bradycardia, junctional rhythm, or second-degree AV block Type I but does not have characteristic signs and symptoms or signs and symptoms subside: Observe the patient.

▼

If the patient has second-degree AV block Type II or third-degree AV block but does not have signs and symptoms or signs and symptoms subside: Insert a transvenous pacemaker.

▼

If the patient has signs and symptoms, regardless of the cause: Administer 0.5 to 1 mg of atropine.

▼

If signs and symptoms persist: Administer 0.5 to 1 mg of atropine and repeat every 5 minutes to a total of 2 mg.

▼

If signs and symptoms still persist: Apply an external pacemaker or administer isoproterenol (2 to 10 mcg/minute) until a transvenous pacemaker can be inserted.

Case study: First- and second-degree AV blocks

Mrs. R., age 68, is admitted to the critical care unit (CCU) with syncope. Having a history of congestive heart failure, she takes 0.25 mg of digoxin (Lanoxin) and 40 mg of furosemide (Lasix) daily, in addition to a potassium supplement. Her weight on admission is 176 lb (80 kg); blood pressure, 130/84 mm Hg; heart rate, 65 beats/minute and regular; respiratory rate, 20 breaths/ minute, with lungs clear on auscultation. Oxygen is administered via nasal cannula at 4 liters/minute. Her rhythm on admission is shown here:

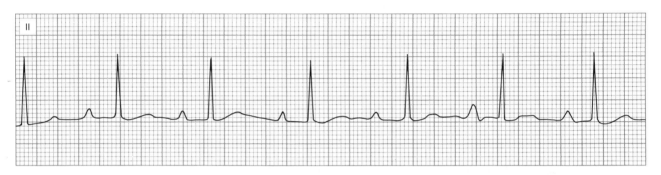

The electrocardiogram (ECG) strip shows sinus rhythm with a first-degree AV block. The PR interval is 0.30 second. In reviewing previous ECG reports, the nurse assigned to Mrs. R. observes that the PR interval has lengthened from an earlier interval of 0.18 second. She notifies Mrs. R.'s physician.

A prolonged PR interval may be caused by a myocardial infarction, ischemia of the AV junction, or toxicity from digoxin, beta blockers, or calcium channel blockers. Most first-degree AV blocks are not treated directly, but the health care team should find and treat the underlying cause, if necessary.

The physician orders laboratory studies to determine Mrs. R.'s digoxin and serum potassium levels. Before the results are available, she exhibits the following rhythm change:

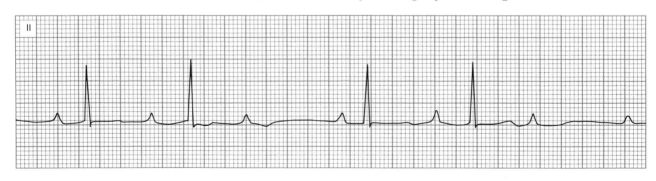

Determine the cause.
Note signs and symptoms.
Administer atropine.

The nurse interprets the rhythm as second-degree AV block Type I (also called Wenckebach or Mobitz I) and checks Mrs. R.'s blood pressure (90/60 mm Hg) and heart rate (50 beats/minute and irregular). Saying she feels light-headed, Mrs. R. becomes increasingly diaphoretic. According to protocol, the nurse administers 0.5 mg of atropine via a heparin lock.

Atropine enhances conduction through the AV node and speeds the heart rate.

Repeat atropine.

The nurse infuses an I.V. solution of dextrose 5% in water at a keep-vein-open rate. After 5 minutes, with no change in Mrs. R.'s rhythm, the nurse administers another 0.5 mg of atropine, which increases the heart rate and triggers the following rhythm change:

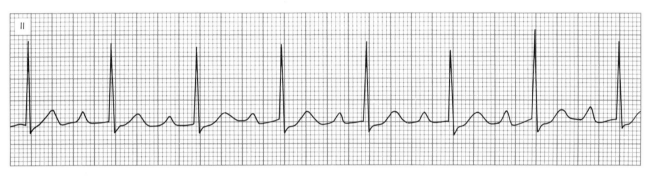

Sinus rhythm with a first-degree AV block returns, matching Mrs. R.'s rhythm on admission with a PR interval of 0.30 second. Her blood pressure is now 110/80 mm Hg; heart rate, 75 beats/minute.

If the first dose of atropine does not achieve the desired effect, additional doses of 0.5 to 1 mg may be administered every 5 minutes, up to a total dose of 2 mg.

Laboratory results on Mrs. R. indicate possible digoxin toxicity. Her digoxin level is 2.6 ng/ml (the therapeutic level is 0.8 to 2 ng/ml). Her potassium level is 3.8 mEq/liter (the normal value is 3.5 to 5 mEq/liter).

Because digoxin has a long half-life (the body excretes it slowly), a patient may require several doses of atropine before the digoxin level in the blood sufficiently decreases. If life-threatening toxicity occurs, a physician may decide to administer digoxin immune FAB (Digibind) or insert a temporary pacemaker. In this case, however, the patient's increased heart rate and the return to sinus rhythm indicate that the digoxin in her blood is approaching a therapeutic level.

Case study: Sinus bradycardia

Mr. G., age 76, is transferred to the hospital's telemetry unit from a skilled nursing facility. Although he experiences left-sided weakness from an earlier cerebrovascular accident, he can ambulate with assistance and usually interacts jovially with caregivers. Just a few days before his transfer, however, nurses at the facility had begun to document his gradually slowing heart rate and atypical lethargy.

Now, a nurse in the telemetry unit records his vital signs: blood pressure, 90/50 mm Hg; heart rate, 30 beats/minute and slightly irregular; respiratory rate, 20 breaths/minute, with rales noted at the lung bases on auscultation. Oxygen is administered at 4 liters/minute by nasal cannula, and the ECG monitor shows the following rhythm:

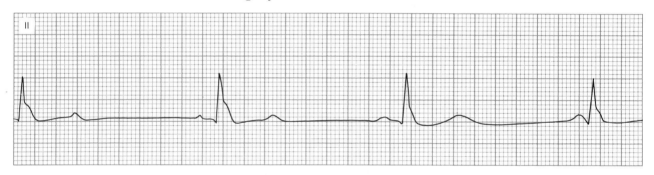

▼ Determine the cause.
Note signs and symptoms.
Administer atropine.

The nurse identifies the rhythm as sinus bradycardia. Although Mr. G.'s heart rate has not varied much with activity since admission, even minimal activity now elicits complaints of chest pain, and his blood pressure has dropped to 84/50 mm Hg. The physician orders 0.5 mg of atropine I.V. The following rhythm appears on the monitor:

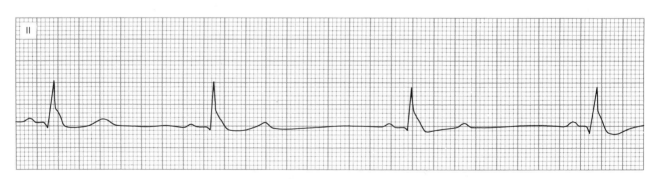

Repeat atropine.

Sinus bradycardia continues. Over the next 10 minutes, with no change in the rhythm, the nurse administers two more 0.5-mg doses of atropine. About 10 minutes after the last dose is given, the nurse notices that Mr. G. has become confused. He seems to be hallucinating and tries to climb out of bed. His rhythm remains unchanged.

If a patient's bradycardia is not caused by increased vagal tone, atropine may prove ineffective in increasing the heart rate. In an elderly patient, the drug can cause confusion or hallucination.

 Insert pacemaker.

The physician concludes that the persistent bradycardia warrants a ventricular pacemaker. Mr. G., whose confusion is abating, maintains a systolic blood pressure of 90 to 96 mm Hg. Because Mr. G. can tolerate the slow rate at rest, the physician decides to implant a permanent pacemaker in the morning and forgo an interim temporary pacemaker. The next day, he inserts a VVI pacemaker, which produces the following rhythm:

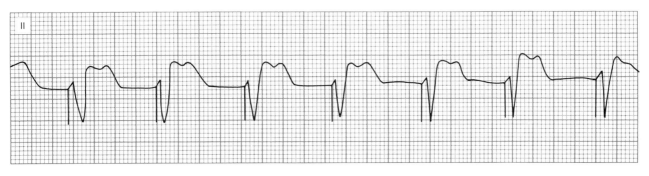

The monitor shows a ventricular-paced rhythm. Mr. G.'s blood pressure is 130/82 mm Hg; his heart rate, 72 beats/minute.

Case study: Junctional escape rhythm

Mr. N., age 64, appears diaphoretic and pale when his daughter brings him into the emergency department (ED). She states that her father has felt chest pains for the past few hours and that the pain has progressively worsened. ED staff members connect Mr. N. to an ECG monitor, which shows sinus bradycardia, and administer oxygen via nasal cannula at 3 liters/minute. A nurse records his blood pressure (148/92 mm Hg), heart rate (54 beats/minute), and respiratory rate (24 breaths/minute, with lungs clear on auscultation). About 10 minutes later, Mr. N.'s rhythm suddenly slows. The low-rate alarm sounds, and the monitor displays the following pattern:

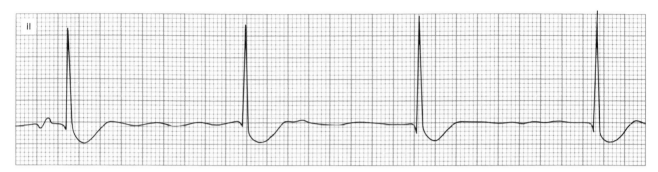

 Determine the cause.

Staff members identify it as junctional escape rhythm.

The beginning of the ECG strip above contains a single P wave in front of the QRS complex; no further P waves appear. Although this backup escape rhythm can sustain a patient, a significant percentage of cardiac output is lost because of the slow rate and the loss of atrial contraction.

 Note signs and symptoms.
Administer atropine.
Repeat atropine.

The nurse rechecks Mr. N.'s blood pressure, which has dropped to 88/54 mm Hg, and heart rate, which has decreased to 35 beats/ minute. As ordered, the nurse administers 0.5 mg of atropine I.V. and, when the first dose has no effect, repeats the dose 5 minutes later. The monitor now shows this rhythm:

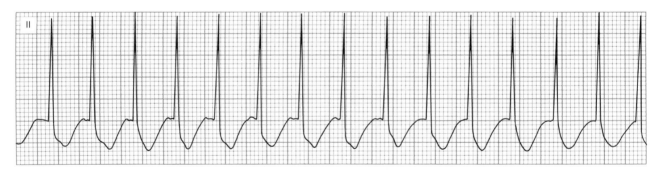

The physician interprets the rhythm as supraventricular tachycardia, possibly junctional. Mr. N.'s blood pressure improves to 100/70 mm Hg. Staff members prepare to transfer him to the CCU for further observation.

Besides increasing the firing rate of the SA node, atropine can enhance automaticity of the AV junction, which may accelerate above the SA node's firing rate and trigger tachycardia. Usually, the arrhythmia slows to a near-normal rate within minutes. In this case, the atropine-triggered tachycardia appears to have improved the patient's blood pressure and probably the cardiac output.

Case study: Third-degree AV block (complete heart block)

Miss M., age 62, is recuperating in the CCU after having an acute anteroseptal myocardial infarction. Weighing about 88 lb (40 kg), she appears alert and well-oriented, and her vital signs are normal (blood pressure, 130/86 mm Hg; heart rate, 70 beats/minute; respiratory rate, 18 breaths/minute). Oxygen is administered via nasal cannula at 3 liters/minute, and she is connected to an ECG monitor, which shows the following rhythm:

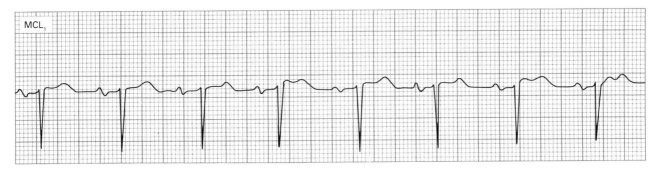

The nurse assigned to Miss M. identifies this as a sinus rhythm, with a rate of 70 to 75 beats/minute. Reviewing ECG reports from earlier in the day, the nurse observes that Miss M. has maintained a normal sinus rhythm, with occasional episodes of sinus tachycardia accompanied by chest pain. A few minutes later, as the nurse prepares to recheck Miss M.'s blood pressure, the low-rate alarm on the ECG monitor sounds, and the following pattern appears:

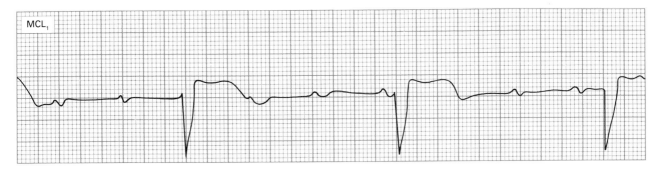

Determine the cause.

The nurse interprets the rhythm as third-degree AV block and notifies Miss M.'s physician, who has just entered the room.

When all supraventricular impulses are prevented from reaching the ventricles, the patient has third-degree AV block (also called complete heart block). In the ECG strip above, note the ventricular escape rhythm that characterizes this condition. The slow rate (30 beats/minute) and the wide QRS complex (0.12 second) indicate that the pacemaking function has been taken over by a ventricular escape rhythm.

 Note signs and symptoms.
Administer atropine.
Repeat atropine.

Miss M.'s blood pressure has decreased to 88/52 mm Hg. She tells the physician that she feels dizzy and complains of heaviness in the chest. The physician directs the nurse to increase the oxygen flow to 5 liters/minute and to administer 0.5 mg of atropine I.V. Miss M.'s rhythm and blood pressure do not improve. About 6 minutes later, the physician orders 1 mg of atropine.

Atropine may not convert a ventricular escape rhythm as effectively as it would a junctional escape rhythm. Thus, a physician may decide to administer 1 mg of atropine for the second dose to reach the full vagolytic dosage rapidly.

 Repeat atropine.
Apply pacemaker.

Miss M.'s rhythm continues. Her heart rate remains about 30 beats/minute. Low blood pressure and chest pain persist. The physician orders an additional 0.5 mg of atropine, but the rhythm does not change, so he decides to use an external pacemaker. He and the nurse place electrodes on Miss M.; then the physician activates the pacemaker, resulting in the following rhythm:

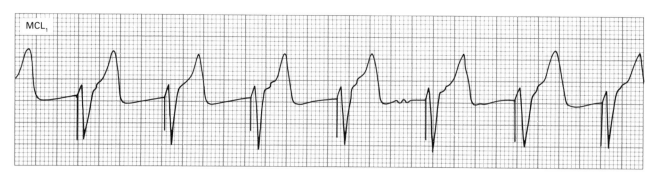

The rhythm indicates successful cardiac pacing, at a rate of 72 beats/minute. Miss M.'s blood pressure has increased to 100/68 mm Hg. She appears to be out of danger. Later, the physician and other CCU staff members will evaluate her for permanent pacemaker insertion.

An external pacemaker can effectively reverse persistent bradycardia until a permanent pacemaker is implanted. As noted in the algorithm, another temporary measure would be to administer isoproterenol (Isuprel) by I.V. drip, titrated to achieve an adequate heart rate. Note, however, that isoproterenol can cause vasodilation, decreased mean arterial pressure, premature ventricular complexes, and increased myocardial oxygen consumption. Considering these possibilities and the patient's chest pain, the physician in the case study elected to use the external pacemaker.

Study questions

Answers to study questions are on page 165.

1. Mr. S., age 46, is admitted to the CCU with a possible inferior wall myocardial infarction. To relieve substernal chest pressure, the physician has ordered 5 mg of morphine sulfate I.V., and Mr. S. is receiving oxygen via nasal cannula at 4 liters/minute. A few minutes earlier, his nurse had recorded his blood pressure (116/80 mm Hg) and, on the ECG monitor, had observed a sinus rhythm, with a rate of 72 beats/minute. Now, however, the nurse notices that the monitor's rate meter shows 45 beats/minute, and the following rhythm appears:

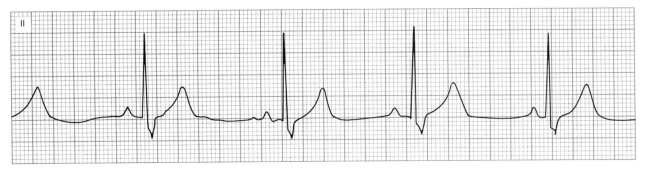

Interpret the rhythm.

2. The nurse rechecks Mr. S.'s vital signs. His blood pressure has decreased to 86/50 mm Hg. His heart rate is 45 beats/minute; respiratory rate, 24 breaths/minute. The nurse observes that Mr. S. seems lethargic. Mr. S. says that his chest pressure has lessened but has not completely gone away. Discuss the next appropriate intervention.

3. Mr. S.'s rhythm continues. What is the next intervention?

4. The ECG monitor now shows this rhythm:

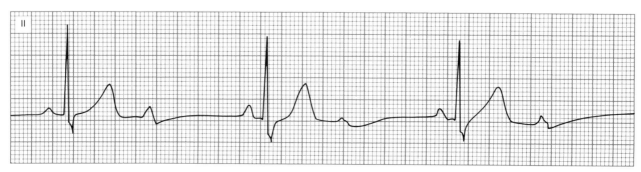

Interpret the rhythm. In your response, explain how you arrived at this interpretation.

5. Within a few minutes, Mr. S.'s rhythm changes again:

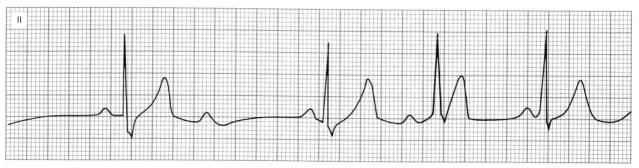

Interpret the rhythm, and estimate Mr. S.'s heart rate based on the last third of the ECG strip.

6. The nurse rechecks Mr. S.'s blood pressure (98/62 mm Hg). Discuss complications for which he should be monitored.

7. Mr. M., age 65, is admitted to the ED after experiencing syncopal episodes that contributed to a minor motor vehicle accident. He has no obvious trauma and tells the admitting nurse that he did not hit his head in the accident. Noting that Mr. M. appears alert and well-oriented, the nurse records his weight (185 lb [84 kg]) and vital signs (blood pressure, 100/72 mm Hg; heart rate, 43 beats/minute; respiratory rate, 22 breaths/minute). ED staff members connect him to an ECG monitor, which shows the following rhythm:

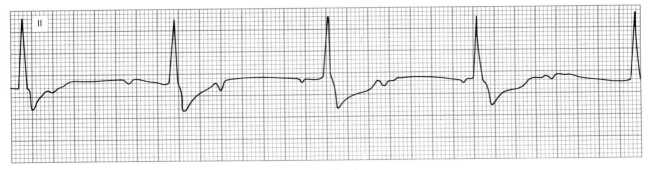

Interpret the rhythm.

8. Mr. M. is no longer complaining of syncope and light-headedness. If these symptoms were to recur, what intervention would the ED physician consider next?

9. State the appropriate intervention if Mr. M. remains free from these symptoms but his rhythm does not change.

Answers to study questions

1. Sinus bradycardia

2. Administer 0.5 mg of atropine I.V. (The low blood pressure indicates that the patient is symptomatic.)

3. Administer another 0.5 mg of atropine I.V.

4. Second-degree AV block Type II. The atrial rate increased from 45 to 65 beats/minute, but now every other P wave is blocked. The PR interval remains constant on conducted beats.

5. The ECG strip shows a change in rhythm from second-degree AV block to sinus bradycardia, with a rate of 56 beats/minute.

6. The patient should be monitored for a recurrence of bradycardia, second- and third-degree AV blocks, and complications from morphine sulfate administration. Patients with inferior wall MI are predisposed to bradycardia and AV blocks. Morphine sulfate, which has a vagomimetic effect, may exacerbate an already slow heart rate.

7. Third-degree AV block (complete heart block)

8. Administer 0.5 mg of atropine I.V.

9. Insert a transvenous pacemaker.

13

Ventricular Ectopy

Ventricular ectopy refers to a condition in which abnormal impulses, called premature ventricular complexes (PVCs), decrease the heart's stroke volume and ventricular filling time, potentially causing inadequate cardiac output, hypotension, and insufficient perfusion of organs. In a patient with myocardial infarction (MI) or ischemia, PVCs may develop into ventricular tachycardia or ventricular fibrillation; acute suppressive drug therapy must be initiated.

The algorithm on the opposite page presents the established emergency treatment protocol for ventricular ectopy. Case studies incorporating the algorithm's interventions follow.

VENTRICULAR ECTOPY

This algorithm presents the emergency measures to take for a patient with ventricular ectopy. Some patients may require interventions not covered in these steps. Before initiating the acute suppressive drug therapy outlined here, the clinician should rule out treatable causes of PVCs: electrolyte imbalances, digoxin toxicity, and bradycardia. The flow of the algorithm presumes that PVCs are continuing. If PVCs resolve after an intervention, follow the maintenance schedule given in parentheses; do not proceed to the next intervention. Note that bretylium may be contraindicated in some patients.

Administer lidocaine (Xylocaine), 1 mg/kg.
(Maintenance: lidocaine drip, 2 mg/minute)
▼
Administer lidocaine, 0.5 mg/kg every 2 to 5 minutes, up to a total dosage of 3 mg/kg.
(Maintenance: lidocaine drip, 3 to 4 mg/minute)
▼
Administer procainamide (Procan), 20 mg/minute, up to a total dosage of 1,000 mg.
(Maintenance: procainamide drip, 1 to 4 mg/minute)
▼
Administer bretylium (Bretylol), 5 to 10 mg/kg over 8 to 10 minutes.
(Maintenance: bretylium drip, 2 mg/minute)
▼
Consider overdrive pacing.

Case study: PVCs caused by ischemia

Mr. S., age 55, is brought to the emergency department (ED) by paramedics. For the past 3 hours, he has felt crushing substernal chest pain that radiates to his jaw. Mr. S. avoided seeking medical attention at first, hoping that rest would relieve the pain. When it intensified, his wife called 911. Now, ED staff members connect him to a cardiac monitor and observe the following rhythm:

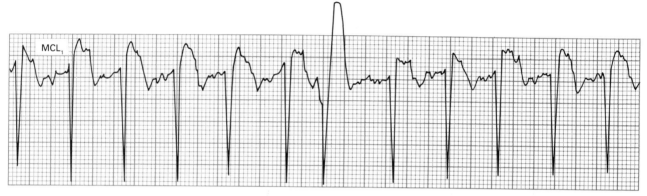

▼ Administer lidocaine.

Identifying the rhythm as sinus tachycardia with one PVC, the ED physician immediately administers lidocaine (Xylocaine), 1 mg/kg.

Lidocaine, a Class IB antiarrhythmic, is the preferred drug for PVCs, ventricular tachycardia, and ventricular fibrillation. Administered prophylactically for suspected MI, lidocaine can effectively suppress PVCs, unstable angina, and certain arrhythmias and prevent the occurrence of more irritable rhythms. Its effects begin in 10 to 90 seconds and last 20 minutes. (See Chapter 5, Pharmacologic Therapy, for more information on lidocaine.)

About 2 minutes later, the following rhythm appears on the monitor:

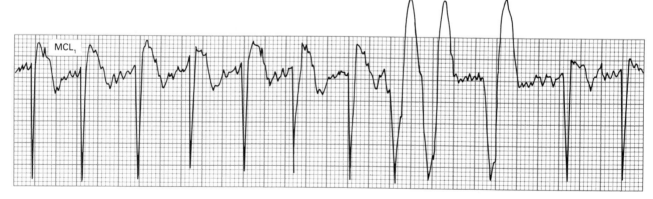

Repeat lidocaine.

Sinus tachycardia continues, with more PVCs apparent. The physician directs a nurse to administer lidocaine, 0.5 mg/kg.

As noted in the algorithm, lidocaine can be repeated every 2 to 5 minutes until PVCs resolve or the maximum dosage of 3 mg/kg is administered.

Now Mr. S.'s rhythm appears as shown:

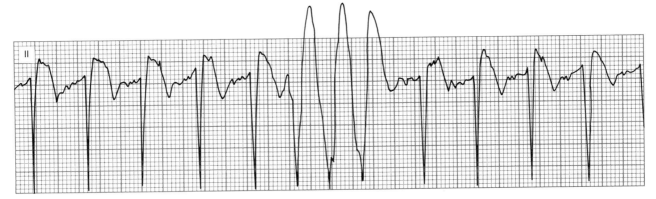

Sinus tachycardia with PVCs continues. Mr. S. is still feeling intense chest pain. One nurse records Mr. S.'s blood pressure (102/ 70 mm Hg), and another administers 2 mg of morphine sulfate by I.V. push, as ordered.

Morphine sulfate, the preferred drug for pain caused by ischemia or infarction, is given intravenously in small doses (usually 2 mg) until pain is relieved. Frequent blood pressure monitoring is critical for two reasons: first, morphine causes vasodilation, which may decrease the patient's blood pressure; second, reduced stroke volume and cardiac output during PVCs may further decrease the blood pressure.

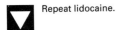 Repeat lidocaine.

Every 2 to 5 minutes, with no change in Mr. S.'s rhythm, the physician orders additional doses of lidocaine until Mr. S. has received the total dosage of 3 mg/kg. The monitor now shows the following rhythm:

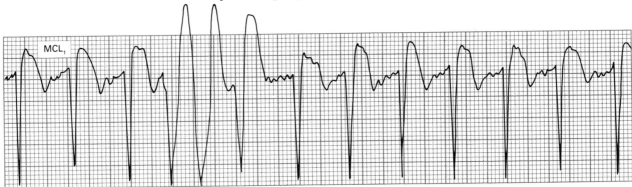

Administer procainamide.

PVCs have not resolved, so the physician orders procainamide (Procan) at 20 mg/minute.

Procainamide, a Class IA antiarrhythmic, is the second-line drug for PVC suppression when lidocaine does not resolve the impulses. Rescuers continue the dosage of 20 mg/minute until the PVCs resolve, the patient becomes hypotensive, the QRS complex widens by at least 50% of its original width, or a total of 1,000 mg has been administered. (See Chapter 5, Pharmacologic Therapy, for more information on procainamide.)

After Mr. S. has received 300 mg of procainamide, the following rhythm appears:

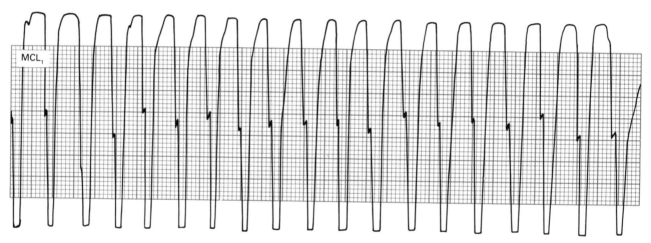

MCL₁

 Treat as VF (see page 85).
Check pulse.
Begin CPR.
Defibrillate with 200 joules.

The physician identifies the rhythm as ventricular tachycardia. The nurse can no longer detect a pulse in Mr. S., and he does not respond when they shake him and call his name. While the nurse calls a Code Blue, the physician begins cardiopulmonary resuscitation (CPR). Code team members arrive and bring a defibrillator to the bedside. The nurse defibrillates the patient with 200 joules.

Pulseless ventricular tachycardia should be treated as ventricular fibrillation (VF) and thus warrants defibrillation. (See the algorithm for VF on page 85. Note that defibrillation should begin even before CPR if a defibrillator is available.)

The following rhythm appears after the first defibrillation attempt:

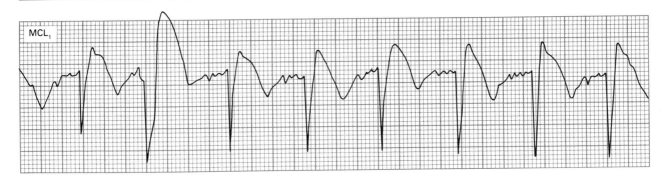

 Administer procainamide (maintenance schedule) after rhythm converts.

Team members recognize this as a sinus rhythm. The nurse can now detect a pulse. The physician orders a procainamide drip at 2 mg/minute and instructs the team to draw a blood sample to determine the serum procainamide level.

After resolution of PVCs or any irritable rhythm, rescuers should start an I.V. infusion to maintain the blood level of the antiarrhythmic drug that eliminated the problem. In this case, because procainamide proved effective, a procainamide infusion of 1 to 4 mg/minute would be the appropriate intervention. The therapeutic blood level of procainamide is 4 to 10 mcg/ml.

Case study: PVCs caused by electrolyte imbalance

Mr. J., age 64, is admitted to the critical care unit (CCU) with an evolving anterior MI and congestive heart failure. Because of the acute MI, the physician administers lidocaine, 1.5 mg/kg by I.V. push, followed by a continuous I.V. infusion of lidocaine at 2 mg/minute.

Many physicians treat patients with acute MI prophylactically to prevent VF. The recommended lidocaine dose for prophylaxis is 1.5 mg/kg followed by an infusion of 2 to 4 mg/minute.

About 10 minutes after the infusion is started, the monitor shows the following rhythm:

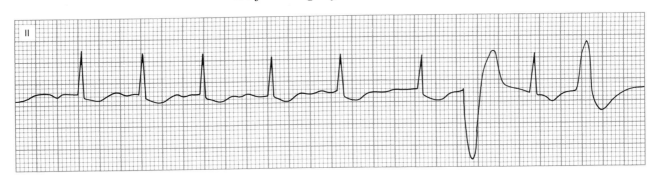

Administer lidocaine.

Observing polymorphic PVCs in the rhythm, the physician orders lidocaine at 1 mg/kg, increases the infusion to 3 mg/minute, and draws venous blood for electrolyte studies.

Polymorphic PVCs (those having different shapes) are usually considered dangerous because they indicate multiple routes of depolarization and multiple ectopic foci. As such, they warrant additional lidocaine therapy. Laboratory studies may reveal an electrolyte imbalance, a possible cause of PVCs.

About 15 minutes later, Mr. J.'s rhythm appears as follows:

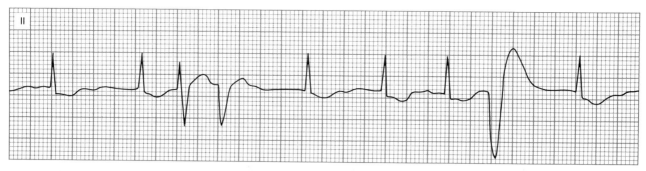

  Repeat lidocaine.

The physician observes continued PVCs with an underlying atrial fibrillation. He orders lidocaine, 0.5 mg/kg, and increases the infusion to 4 mg/minute. Laboratory studies indicate that Mr. J.'s electrolyte levels are within normal range, except for a potassium level of 3 mEq/liter (the normal value is 3.5 to 5 mEq/liter). As ordered, the nurse adds 40 mEq of potassium to 100 ml of dextrose 5% in water, to be infused over 1 hour.

Whenever PVCs occur, consider an electrolyte imbalance, such as hyperkalemia or hypokalemia, as a possible cause. Potassium affects the electrical activity of all muscle, including the myocardium. In the case study, the patient's hypokalemia probably resulted from administration of a diuretic to treat congestive heart failure. Other possible causes of PVCs include digoxin toxicity, bradycardia, hypoxemia, hypercapnia, ischemia, excitement, pain, and excessive caffeine or nicotine intake.

About 10 minutes have elapsed since the potassium infusion was started. On the ECG monitor, the physician observes the following rhythm:

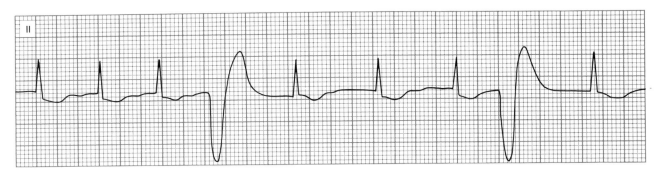

Atrial fibrillation continues, with PVCs still apparent. Mr. J.'s blood pressure is 116/82 mm Hg. He tells the physician that he is not feeling chest pain.

Recurrent PVCs can cause incomplete ventricular filling. When this happens, stroke volume and cardiac output subsequently decrease, and the resultant myocardial ischemia can produce abrupt chest pain.

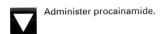
Administer procainamide.

Because PVCs continue and Mr. J. has received the maximum dosage of lidocaine (3 mg/kg), the physician orders procainamide, 20 mg/minute, by slow I.V. push. After 200 mg have been administered, the following rhythm appears:

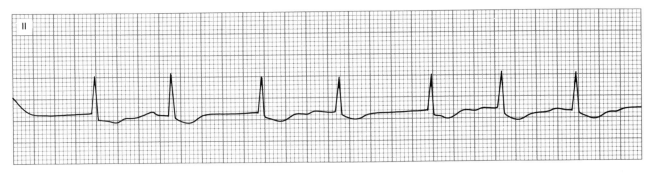

Although atrial fibrillation continues, the PVCs have resolved. Mr. J.'s blood pressure is 118/80 mm Hg. He remains free from chest pain.

As noted earlier, procainamide administration is the recommended intervention when lidocaine fails to suppress PVCs. The dosage is 20 mg/minute until PVCs resolve, hypotension occurs, the QRS complex widens by at least 50% of its original width, or a total of 1,000 mg has been infused.

The physician orders a procainamide infusion at 1 mg/minute and draws another sample of Mr. J.'s blood for laboratory analysis of electrolyte and serum procainamide levels.

Administer procainamide (maintenance schedule).

When PVCs resolve, the appropriate intervention is to begin infusing the drug that corrected the problem. The recommended infusion rate for procainamide is 1 to 4 mg/minute. Laboratory analysis of the patient's blood will reveal his serum procainamide level (the therapeutic level is 4 to 10 mcg/ml) and confirm whether potassium administration has corrected the electrolyte imbalance.

Case study: PVCs caused by digoxin toxicity

Mrs. G., age 80, schedules an appointment with her family physician because she "feels like my heart is skipping beats." She has a history of MI and congestive heart failure but has been stable recently, experiencing no anginal pain. Her medication regimen includes 0.25 mg of digoxin (Lanoxin) daily, 375 mg of procainamide every 6 hours, 20 mg of furosemide (Lasix) every other day, and 1 tablet of potassium each morning. At the physician's office, a nurse records Mrs. G.'s blood pressure (90/55 mm Hg), which has decreased since the last office visit (122/80 mm Hg). Mrs. G. tells the physician that she feels dizzy. He connects her to an ECG monitor, which shows the following rhythm:

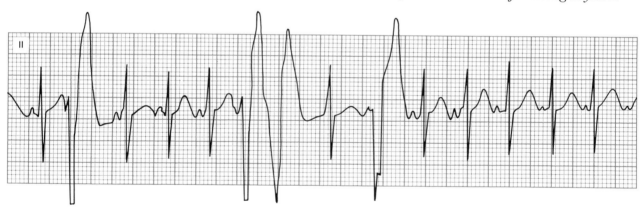

Identifying the rhythm as sinus tachycardia with PVCs, the physician arranges for an ambulance to take Mrs. G. to the ED for assessment and treatment.

PVCs are especially significant in this case because the patient's history of MI suggests the possibility of ischemic PVCs and extension of MI. Furthermore, the low blood pressure and dizziness indicate decreased cardiac output, which may be associated with extension of MI or cardiac failure.

 Administer lidocaine.

In the ED, a nurse draws a blood sample for laboratory analysis to determine Mrs. G.'s serum potassium, digoxin, and procainamide levels, and the physician orders lidocaine 1 mg/kg by I.V. push.

While instituting suppressive drug therapy for PVCs as outlined in the algorithm, the clinician should rule out all treatable causes of PVCs, such as an electrolyte imbalance, drug toxicity, or bradycardia. For bradycardia associated with PVCs, atropine (rather than lidocaine or procainamide) is usually administered to increase the heart rate and suppress the PVCs. In this case, the patient's rapid heart rate warrants treatment with lidocaine, a cardiac depressant.

About 2 minutes after administering the lidocaine, the nurse observes the following rhythm on the monitor:

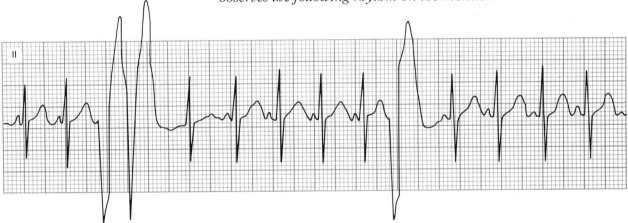

Repeat lidocaine.

Administer bretylium.

Sinus tachycardia continues, with PVCs still apparent. Every 2 minutes, the nurse administers another dose of lidocaine, 0.5 mg/ kg, until Mrs. G. has received the maximum recommended dosage of 3 mg/kg, but her rhythm does not change. Her blood pressure of 98/60 mm Hg has improved only slightly since admission. She is not feeling chest pain. Laboratory studies reveal normal electrolyte levels, a digoxin level of 2.8 ng/ml (the therapeutic level is 1 to 2 ng/ml), and a procainamide level of 10 mg/ml (the therapeutic level is 4 to 10 mg/ml). The physician orders bretylium (Bretylol), 5 mg/kg, to be infused slowly over 8 minutes.

At this point, the physician must consider several factors. The abnormally high digoxin level is probably causing the PVCs (although electrolyte imbalances can potentiate digoxin toxicity, this patient's electrolyte levels are normal). Because PVCs are continuing and the patient's blood pressure remains low, acute suppressive drug therapy is necessary. However, the physician has already administered the maximum lidocaine dosage, and the patient's high procainamide level nearly exceeds the normal range, making procainamide administration risky. Therefore, the physician decides to administer bretylium, even though the drug works slowly and may produce hypotension, nausea, and vomiting.

About 15 minutes after he administers the bretylium, the physician observes the following rhythm on the monitor:

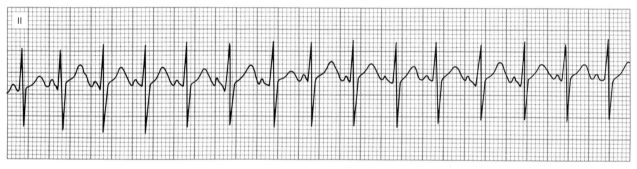

▼ Administer bretylium (maintenance schedule).

Although sinus tachycardia continues, the PVCs have resolved. The physician orders a bretylium infusion at 2 mg/minute. Mrs. G.'s blood pressure has improved to 110/74 mm Hg. ED staff members prepare to transfer her to the CCU for further observation and treatment.

As noted in the algorithm, once PVCs resolve, the appropriate intervention is to begin infusing the drug that corrected the problem. The recommended maintenance dose for bretylium is 2 mg/kg. If maximum dosages of lidocaine, procainamide, and bretylium fail to suppress PVCs, a physician may try overdrive cardiac pacing (which was not necessary in this case). Overdrive pacing—ventricular pacing that is faster than the patient's intrinsic rate—may break the impulse conduction pattern that characterizes PVCs. (See Chapter 6, Electrical and Mechanical Interventions, for a more detailed discussion of pacemaker therapy.)

Study questions

Answers to study questions are on pages 180 and 181.

1. Responding to a 911 call, paramedics arrive at the home of Mr. J., who has taken several nitroglycerin tablets for crushing substernal chest pain that continues to radiate to his left shoulder and arm. The paramedics record Mr. J.'s blood pressure (98/60 mm Hg), heart rate (112 beats/minute), and respiratory rate (22 breaths/minute) and connect him to an ECG monitor, which shows the following rhythm:

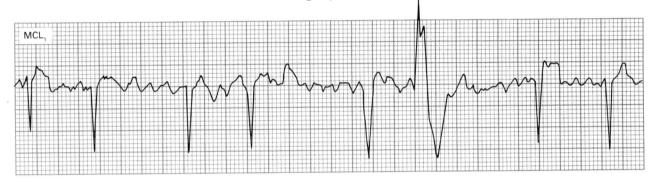

   Interpret the rhythm.

2. Name three appropriate interventions for the paramedics to consider before transporting Mr. J. to the hospital.

3. The paramedics take Mr. J. into the ED, reporting that they have administered lidocaine at a total dose of 2.5 mg/kg. The ECG monitor now shows the following rhythm:

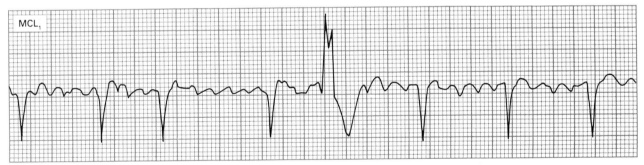

   ED staff members identify the rhythm as atrial fibrillation, with flutter waves and PVCs apparent. Mr. J.'s blood pressure is 96/50 mm Hg, and he still complains of severe chest pain. Identify the next two interventions.

4. What is the maximum recommended lidocaine dosage for PVCs?

5. PVCs are still apparent in Mr. J.'s rhythm. What is probably causing them?

6. Name the next appropriate intervention.

7. What is the maximum recommended procainamide dosage for PVCs?

8. After 300 mg of procainamide have been administered, Mr. J.'s rhythm appears as follows:

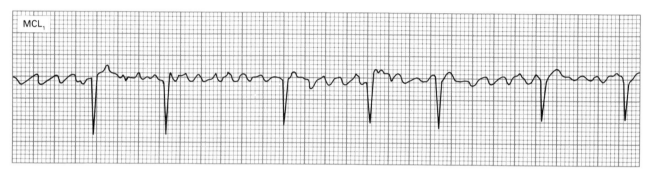

The physician recognizes this as atrial fibrillation with flutter waves. PVCs have resolved. What should the physician do next?

9. Staff members are preparing to transfer Mr. J. to the CCU. Which blood tests should the physician order?

10. Mr. G., age 56, is admitted to the CCU with an acute anterior wall MI. Because of this diagnosis, the physician administers lidocaine 1.5 mg/kg prophylactically. The next day, Mr. G.'s nurse observes the following rhythm on the monitor:

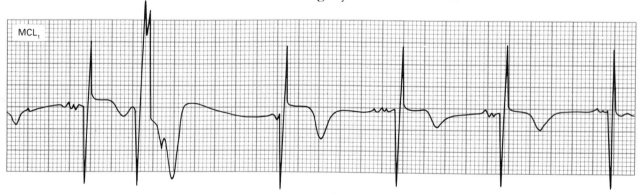

Identify the rhythm.

11. Which interventions are appropriate in response to this rhythm?

12. After Mr. G. has received lidocaine, 3 mg/kg, his rhythm appears as follows:

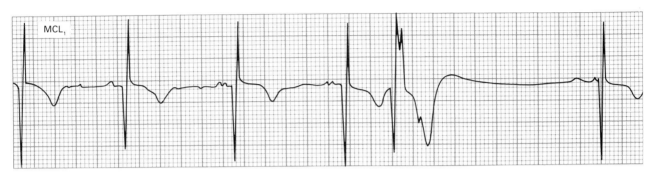

Identify the rhythm.

13. Discuss the appropriate intervention for this rhythm.

14. The physician decides to administer procainamide. After 100 mg have been administered, Mr. G.'s rhythm remains unchanged, and his blood pressure is 80/50 mm Hg. What should the physician do next?

15. Mr. G. is receiving bretylium at 5 mg/kg when the following rhythm appears:

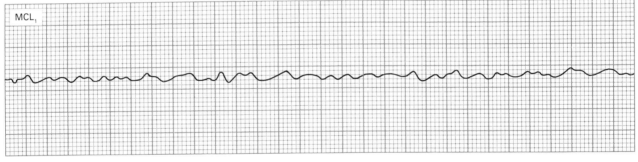

Identify the rhythm.

16. Name appropriate interventions in response to this rhythm.

17. After the last intervention, a sinus rhythm appears on the monitor. Mr. G. has a strong pulse and is breathing spontaneously. Identify the next intervention, and explain its purpose.

18. Mr. B., age 59, is admitted to the ED for chest pain and shortness of breath that began 4 hours ago. His history includes an anterior wall MI (3 years ago) and coronary artery angioplasty (6 months

ago). He appears diaphoretic as a nurse records his blood pressure (98/58 mm Hg), heart rate (66 beats/minute), and respiratory rate (26 breaths/minute, with bibasilar rales on auscultation). ED staff members connect him to an ECG monitor, which shows the following rhythm:

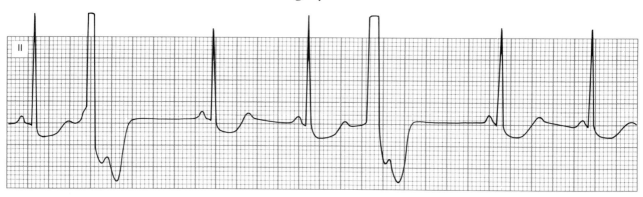

Identify the rhythm.

19. Name the first appropriate intervention in response to this rhythm.

Answers to study questions

1. Atrial fibrillation with flutter waves

2. Administer oxygen, establish an I.V. line, and administer lidocaine, 1 mg/kg.

3. Administer medication to relieve the pain (usually, morphine sulfate I.V., 2 mg every 5 minutes, not to exceed 10 mg/hour), and administer lidocaine, 0.5 mg/kg I.V.

4. 3 mg/kg

5. Ischemia

6. Administer procainamide, 20 mg/minute.

7. 1,000 mg

8. Infuse procainamide I.V. at 1 to 4 mg/minute.

9. The physician should order blood drawn to determine the patient's serum procainamide level, electrolyte levels, and arterial blood gas values. (Although not discussed in the case, the physician may also order cardiac enzyme studies to evaluate the possibility of MI.)

10. Sinus rhythm with one PVC

11. First, administer lidocaine at 1 mg/kg. If PVCs continue, administer 0.5 mg/kg every 2 to 5 minutes until PVCs resolve or the patient has received 3 mg/kg, the maximum recommended dosage.

12. Sinus rhythm with continued PVCs

13. Administer procainamide, 20 mg/minute I.V.

14. Discontinue the procainamide, and administer bretylium 5 to 10 mg/kg over 8 to 10 minutes. (Remember, procainamide can produce hypotension. If this develops, rescuers must discontinue the drug.)

15. Ventricular fibrillation

16. Check the patient for a pulse. Determine whether he responds to gentle shaking or verbal stimuli. If he is pulseless and unresponsive, begin CPR and defibrillate as soon as possible.

17. Begin a bretylium infusion at 2 mg/minute to prevent the arrhythmia from recurring.

18. Sinus rhythm with PVCs

19. Administer lidocaine, 1 mg/kg.

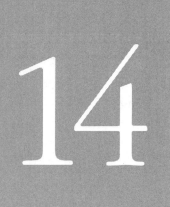

14

Pediatric Emergencies

Although cardiac arrest in children can result from diverse conditions, the emergency typically originates in the respiratory or circulatory system and is usually associated with profound hypoxemia and acidosis. A primary cardiac event in children is relatively rare. Thus, this chapter focuses on anticipatory assessment and intervention, emphasizing adequate ventilation to prevent hypoxemia and respiratory acidosis. Case studies highlight three of the most common cardio-pulmonary pediatric emergencies.

Case study: Respiratory distress

Luke R., age 4, is brought to the emergency department (ED) by his mother for treatment of a severe sore throat and cough. A nurse records his weight (33 lb [15 kg]) and vital signs. After a brief examination, the ED physician instructs the nurse to collect a throat culture specimen and then discharges Luke, prescribing antibiotics pending results of the throat culture. The next morning, Luke's mother brings him back to the ED, stating that he has had a fever and increasing difficulty breathing through the night. Assessment demonstrates inspiratory stridor and wheezing throughout the lung fields, severe dyspnea, a respiratory rate of 52 breaths/ minute, and inspiratory retractions. The physician connects Luke to an electrocardiogram (ECG) monitor and observes the following rhythm:

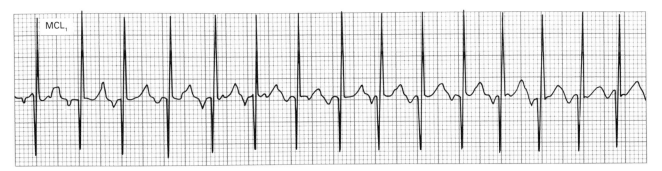

The physician identifies the rhythm as supraventricular tachycardia, noting that Luke's heart rate is greater than 150 beats/minute.

Inspiratory retractions, an increased respiratory rate, tachycardia, and respiratory distress indicate a compensatory state in which the patient can maintain oxygenation only with extreme respiratory effort. This lasts until the patient, exhausted, can no longer breathe independently. Respiratory failure will ensue unless clinicians intervene appropriately to treat respiratory distress. Because a pediatric patient's airway is smaller and supported by less cartilage than that of an adult, it can easily become obstructed by mucus, edema, or constriction. All three of these are probably contributing to the patient's condition in this case study.

The physician directs a nurse to draw blood for arterial blood gas (ABG) studies and begins administering oxygen by face tent at 40% (0.4 FIO_2).

In this case, the patient's condition warranted immediate oxygen support, even before ABG results would be available. A face tent is sometimes used to administer oxygen in pediatric emergencies because children tolerate it better than a face mask. The face tent can deliver high concentrations of oxygen (greater than 50%) with high oxygen flow, although maintaining a high concentration can be difficult because room air enters during patient care. Another advantage of the face tent is that, unlike a nasal cannula, it permits humidification.

Laboratory analysis yields the following ABG values: pH, 7.22; Pco₂, 60 mm Hg; Po₂, 45 mm Hg; HCO₃, 24 mEq/liter; O₂ saturation, 78%. The physician diagnoses respiratory acidosis (low pH, high Pco₂) and hypoxemia (the Po₂ is less than 60 mm Hg). Respiratory distress, inspiratory retractions, and labored breathing continue, and Luke now demonstrates nasal flaring. He is pale and cyanotic around the mouth. His respiratory rate has increased to 64 breaths/minute. The physician directs ED staff to prepare Luke for intubation. They insert an I.V. line.

The patient's ABG values and labored breathing indicate respiratory failure, which warrants intubation. For I.V. cannulation, the staff should use the largest and most accessible vein. Usually, central vein cannulation is preferred because it allows the use of a larger cannula and affords a more direct route for drug administration.

A nurse rechecks Luke's vital signs, noting that his heart rate has decreased to 100 beats/minute. On the ECG monitor, the following rhythm appears:

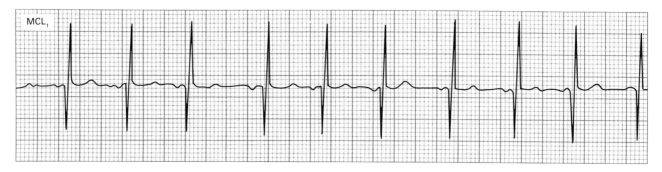

The nurse identifies the rhythm as sinus tachycardia. Luke's heart rate continues to decrease. The physician immediately orders oxygen administration at 100% by face mask.

In an adult, a heart rate of less than 100 beats/minute is normal. When a pediatric patient's heart rate slows to less than 100 beats/minute, however, the staff must identify the cause and intervene appropriately.

A slow heart rate in a pediatric patient usually results from atrioventricular (AV) block, excess vagal tone, or suppression of normal cardiac electrical activity caused by acidosis and hypoxemia. In this case, hypoxemia is probably causing the slow heart rate, so oxygen administration is the appropriate intervention.

On the ECG monitor, the physician observes the following rhythm:

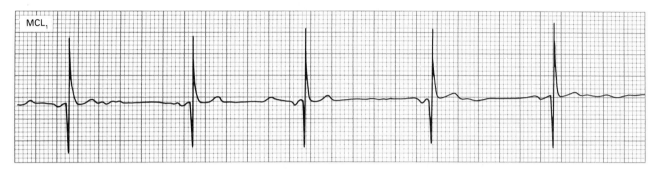

Identifying this as a sinus rhythm, the physician immediately intubates Luke and continues oxygen at 100% by manual resuscitation bag. The nurse states that Luke's heart rate has decreased to about 50 beats/minute.

Intubation promotes adequate ventilation and oxygenation. After intubation, the team should auscultate all lung fields while ventilating the patient with a manual resuscitation bag. (If team members can detect lung sounds in all lung fields, the endotracheal tube has been positioned properly. Once the patient is stable, a chest X-ray should be ordered to confirm the tube's positioning.) Heart rate should always be monitored during intubation of a young child because mechanical stimulation of the airway may induce reflex bradycardia, a sign of hypoxemia. *Note:* Although not done in this case, atropine (0.02 mg/kg) is sometimes administered before intubation to prevent hypoxemia-induced bradycardia.

Suddenly, Luke's rhythm changes to the following:

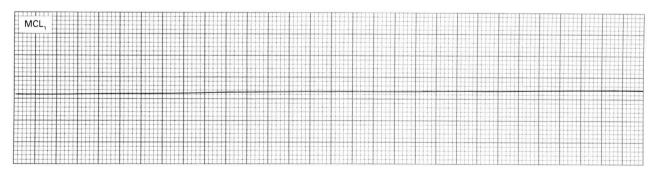

The physician identifies the rhythm as asystole. The nurse, announcing that Luke has no pulse or respirations, changes the monitor leads to recheck the rhythm in a second lead, confirms asystole, and calls a code as the physician begins cardiopulmonary resuscitation (CPR).

Characterized by lack of a palpable pulse and respirations, asystole warrants immediate basic life support measures. The algorithm for asystole on page 115 should be used for children as well as for adults. Although the team's interventions to prevent asystole in this case have been prompt and appropriate, cardiac tissue hypoxia had probably progressed sufficiently to cause cardiac arrest. The patient was also at higher risk for asystole because a child's metabolic rate is twice that of an adult (oxygen consumption is 6 to 8 ml/kg/minute in a child, 3 to 4 ml/kg/minute in an adult). With inadequate ventilation or gas exchange, hypoxemia and subsequent tissue hypoxia occur rapidly.

As other code team members arrive, the physician orders blood drawn for a serum glucose level and ABG analysis.

A pediatric patient has limited glycogen stores that, if depleted rapidly, can induce hypoglycemia. Because clinical signs of hypoglycemia (tachycardia, altered level of consciousness, weak pulse, bradycardia, and hypotension) can mimic those of hypoxemia, determining the patient's serum glucose level is advisable. Anaerobic metabolism induced by hypoxemia yields lactic acid that, in combination with respiratory failure, causes respiratory and metabolic acidosis. ABG analysis can help determine the severity of the problem. Respiratory acidosis is usually corrected by improving ventilation.

The physician administers epinephrine (Adrenalin), 0.01 mg/kg of a 1:10,000 I.V. solution.

Epinephrine is administered for asystole and certain bradyarrhythmias to stimulate cardiac electrical and mechanical activity.

Laboratory results indicate that Luke's serum glucose level is 48 mg/dl (the normal level is 80 to 120 mg/dl). The physician orders 30 ml of dextrose 50% in water ($D_{50}W$), diluted in sterile water in a 1:4 ratio.

Strong myocardial contraction may depend on adequate serum glucose levels. The recommended glucose dose is 0.5 to 1 g/kg. The child weighs 15 kg, and the physician orders the nurse to administer the maximum dose. Since glucose is available as $D_{50}W$ (0.5 g/ml), the nurse must administer 30 ml (15 g) of the available solution, diluted in a 1:4 ratio with sterile water because the hyperosmolarity of the $D_{50}W$ could have a sclerosing effect on the veins.

CPR continues. About 5 minutes after the patient has received epinephrine, the following rhythm appears:

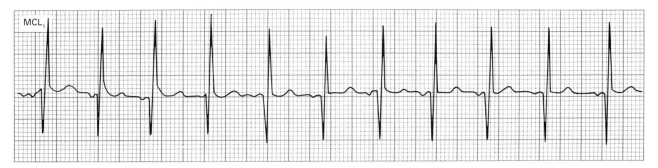

The physician identifies the rhythm as sinus tachycardia. The nurse detects peripheral pulses. Luke's blood pressure is 106/64 mm Hg; his heart rate, 140 beats/minute. Staff members prepare to transfer him to the pediatric intensive care unit (PICU) for further observation and treatment.

Case study: Paroxysmal supraventricular tachycardia

Kevin J., age 6, is brought to the ED by his parents after experiencing dizziness, light-headedness, weakness, and confusion. Medical records indicate that Kevin, who weighs 55 lb [25 kg], has an accessory conduction pathway. The ED physician connects him to an ECG monitor, which shows the following rhythm:

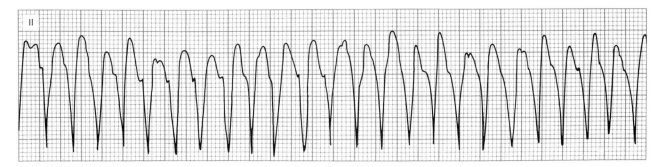

The physician identifies the rhythm as paroxysmal supraventricular tachycardia (PSVT), with a ventricular rate of 220 beats/minute.

The rapid ventricular rate decreases diastolic filling time, thus producing the patient's symptoms. Some individuals are born with an abnormal electrical conduction pathway that parallels the AV junction. This accessory pathway does not have the usual conduction delay associated with the AV node. Thus, impulses travel more rapidly through it than through the AV node. Early stimulation of the ventricle accounts for preexcitation syndromes. The most common type of accessory pathway is the Kent bundle. (See Chapter 3, The 12-Lead ECG, for more information about accessory pathways and preexcitation syndromes.)

The physician asks the nurse to start an I.V. line and administer oxygen at 4 liters/minute by nasal cannula.

Drug administration is always a possibility when treating an arrhythmia. Establishing an I.V. line permits the team to administer medications quickly in an emergency. Oxygen administration helps prevent hypoxemia and tissue hypoxia, which can develop because PSVT increases myocardial oxygen demand and decreases filling time and stroke volume.

A nurse records Kevin's blood pressure (78/50 mm Hg), noting that he appears lethargic. His peripheral pulses are barely palpable, and his capillary refill time is 5 seconds. The physician orders oxygen administration at 40% by face mask and instructs the staff to prepare for cardioversion.

Treatment of an asymptomatic child with PSVT usually consists only of oxygen administration, and the child is observed for spontaneous conversion. However, this patient's weak peripheral pulses and slow capillary refill time indicate decreased cardiac output, a condition that warrants more aggressive treatment.

The physician institutes cardioversion at 25 joules, and the following rhythm appears on the monitor:

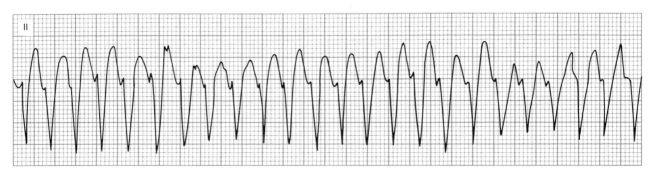

PSVT continues, so the physician attempts cardioversion again, this time using 50 joules.

Cardioversion is the recommended treatment for supraventricular tachycardia associated with cardiovascular instability (evidenced by weak peripheral pulses and slow capillary refill time). The treatment goal is to depolarize a critical mass of myocardial cells and break the tachycardic pattern. The recommended energy level for the first cardioversion attempt is 0.5 to 1 joule/kg; for the second attempt, 2 joules/kg.

After the second attempt, the following rhythm appears:

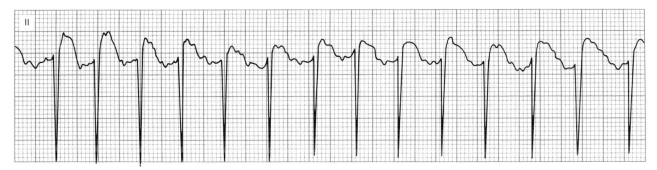

The physician identifies the rhythm as sinus tachycardia. Now able to palpate Kevin's pulse, the nurse states that his blood pressure has improved to 105/65 mm Hg. After cardiac output increases and Kevin's condition stabilizes, staff members transfer him to the PICU, where he is scheduled for electrophysiologic study to evaluate his accessory pathway.

Case study: Hypovolemia

Sara H., age 7, is brought to the ED by her mother, who states that Sara has had diarrhea and a poor appetite for 5 days. A nurse records Sara's weight (55 lb [25 kg]) and vital signs (blood pressure, 102/68 mm Hg; heart rate, 150 beats/minute; respiratory rate, 36 breaths/minute) before connecting her to an ECG monitor, which shows the following rhythm:

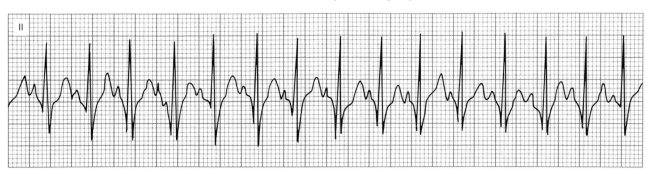

Interpreting the rhythm as sinus tachycardia, the nurse immediately notifies the ED physician, who arrives to examine the child. He observes that Sara's peripheral pulses are weak and her skin is pale and cool to the touch. Sara's mother states that her daughter has not urinated since morning, about 8 hours earlier.

Hypovolemic shock, a common problem in pediatric patients, can result from trauma, burns, or diabetic ketoacidosis but also may be associated with dehydration following diarrhea, vomiting, or decreased appetite. In infants and children, the condition is considered an emergency because they have less fluid reserves than adults do. Fluid losses from diarrhea and vomiting are more likely to cause shock symptoms, such as decreased tissue perfusion. Blood pressure is not a reliable indicator of hypovolemic shock in children. Heart rate, urine output, skin color and temperature, and amplitude of peripheral pulses are more reliable. Hypotension can be a late sign of cardiovascular failure in children.

The physician inserts a 14-cm I.V. cannula in the superior vena cava via the subclavian vein.

Because the patient requires fluid administration, establishing an I.V. line is vital, preferably using the largest and most easily accessible vein. A central vein enables the clinician to use a larger cannula and provides the most direct route for administration. Additionally, fluids administered through a large cannula in a large vein are easier for the patient to tolerate.

Next, the nurse administers oxygen through a nasal cannula at 2 liters/minute.

Although the patient does not appear to have respiratory difficulty at this time, oxygen is administered to help prevent hypoxemia and tissue hypoxia. The staff should administer oxygen in the least invasive, most comfortable way possible (such as nasal cannula) unless signs of respiratory distress—increased respiratory rate, inspiratory retractions, dyspnea, nasal flaring, and cyanosis—dictate otherwise.

The physician then orders an infusion of lactated Ringer's solution, at 20 ml/kg.

Fluid replacement usually begins with a crystalloid solution, such as lactated Ringer's, to expand interstitial water space and correct sodium deficits. The usual dose is 20 ml/kg, infused rapidly for about 20 minutes. Colloid solutions and blood products, more effective in expanding the intravascular compartment, are administered as soon as possible after that. Unless the patient has hypoglycemia, dextrose solutions are not used because the possible resultant hyperglycemia may cause osmotic diuresis and further fluid volume loss.

Sara's skin remains pale and cool, her peripheral pulses weak. The physician inserts an indwelling urinary catheter and orders 250 ml of normal serum albumin 5%.

Albumin increases osmotic pressure in the vessels and intravascular volume. The usual dose is 10 ml/kg. Indwelling catheter insertion helps facilitate accurate calculation of urine output.

Sara's skin remains cool and damp after the albumin administration, and her urine is very concentrated. The physician orders normal saline solution, 20 ml/kg, to be infused over the next 20 minutes.

Hypovolemic shock results from decreased intravascular and extravascular fluid volume. As the condition worsens, capillaries become more permeable and leak fluid. Because of this additional fluid loss, the volume of fluid replaced should be greater than the estimated loss. In this case, the physician is guarding against inadequate fluid volume replacement, a common risk with pediatric patients. Hypovolemic shock in a child may warrant 40 to 60 ml/kg during the first hour and 100 to 200 ml/kg in the first few hours. The recommended procedure is to administer a bolus of fluid and then reassess the patient. Successful treatment of hypovolemia depends on frequent assessment and adequate fluid replacement.

About 20 minutes after beginning the infusion of normal saline solution, the physician and the nurse reassess Sara's condition. Although sinus tachycardia continues, her heart rate has decreased to 110 beats/minute, her pulse is stronger, and skin color and temperature have improved. The physician admits Sara to the pediatric unit for continued fluid therapy and stabilization.

Study questions

Answers to study questions are on pages 193 and 194.

1. Ben E., age 8, is brought to the ED by his parents, who tell the admitting nurse that he has had nausea and vomiting for 2 days, has been unable to keep food or fluids down, and has had diarrhea for about 5 days. Ben weighs 66 lb [30 kg]. Which assessments should the ED staff make?

2. Which condition does Ben probably have?

3. Name the first two interventions the ED staff should consider to treat this condition.

4. Ben's condition worsens. He has dry mucous membranes and poor skin turgor. His heart rate is 158 beats/minute; respiratory rate, 42 breaths/minute; and blood pressure, 108/62 mm Hg. He is confused and does not recognize his parents. What kind of fluid should the staff administer?

5. How much fluid should they administer?

6. Staff members regularly assess Ben's condition for signs of improvement. Name several signs that would indicate adequate fluid replacement.

7. Jessica T., age 2, has had a cold and an ear infection for 4 days. Antibiotics prescribed by her pediatrician have not improved her condition. Her mother brings her to the ED after Jessica exhibits worsening shortness of breath, coughing, and audible wheezing. She states that a humidifier in Jessica's room has not helped. Which assessments should the ED staff make?

8. What are the major concerns?

9. Staff members note audible wheezing, decreased breath sounds, and substernal and intercostal retractions. Jessica is restless and irritable. Name the next three interventions the staff should perform.

10. Further assessment reveals that Jessica's condition is worsening. Which signs might indicate this to the staff?

11. ABG analysis yields these results: pH, 7.28; Po_2, 52 mm Hg; Pco_2, 62 mm Hg; HCO_3, 18 mEq/liter; O_2 saturation, 76%. How would you interpret the results?

12. Discuss what the ED staff should do next.

13. Instructing the staff to prepare for endotracheal intubation, the physician orders atropine, 0.02 mg/kg I.V. What is the rationale for atropine administration?

14. After the physician administers atropine and completes endotracheal intubation, Jessica stabilizes, and she appears out of danger. What is the physician likely to do next?

Answers to study questions

1. The staff should assess the patient's vital signs, neurologic status (dizziness and confusion), cardiovascular status (peripheral pulses, heart rate, skin color and temperature), and urine output (for evidence of renal perfusion).

2. The patient probably has hypovolemia.

3. To treat hypovolemia, the staff should establish an I.V. line and begin fluid replacement.

4. The staff should administer a crystalloid solution, probably lactated Ringer's or normal saline.

5. The recommended dose is 20 ml/kg, infused over 20 to 30 minutes. For this patient, who weighs 30 kg, the appropriate dose would be 600 ml.

6. Palpable peripheral pulses, recognition of parents, increased urine output with decreased urine concentration, and decreased heart rate would suggest adequate fluid replacement.

7. The staff should assess the patient's lungs (for crackles, rhonchi, and air movement in all lung fields), respiratory rate, skin color and temperature, heart rate, and level of consciousness. The staff should also observe the patient for use of accessory muscles (abdominal and shoulder), which would indicate respiratory distress.

8. Hypoxemia and respiratory failure

9. Staff members should administer oxygen (by face tent or face mask, whichever is better tolerated), obtain blood specimens (for ABG analysis and to determine the patient's serum glucose level), and establish an I.V. line.

10. Stridor, grunting, a respiratory rate greater than 60 breaths/minute, a heart rate greater than 180 beats/minute or less than 80 beats/minute, and inability of the patient to recognize her parents suggest a worsening condition.

11. The ABG results indicate combined respiratory and metabolic acidosis. With moderate hypoxemia, oxygen saturation will be decreased.

12. To manage the patient's acidosis and hypoxemia and to prevent cardiac arrest, the staff should try to improve the patient's ventilation. Even the metabolic acidosis is treated with hyperventilation to decrease CO_2. Sodium bicarbonate administration may be considered only if cardiac arrest and acidosis persist after the patient's airway has been secured, the patient has been hyperventilated, the staff is performing chest compressions, and epinephrine has been administered.

13. Atropine administration can help reduce incidence of brady-arrhythmia during intubation.

14. Because the patient is stable and appears out of danger, the physician will probably transfer her to the PICU for further observation and treatment.

Appendix

Self-Test

Take this self-test to evaluate your understanding of the material presented in Chapters 1 to 14. The test consists of brief scenarios with clinical information, electrocardiogram (ECG) monitor recordings for interpretation, and pertinent questions about appropriate interventions. Answers to the self-test are on pages 205 to 209.

1. Mr. G., age 60, is admitted to the emergency department (ED) for treatment of substernal chest pain, nausea, and profuse diaphoresis. A nurse records his weight (154 lb [70 kg]) and vital signs (blood pressure, 110/74 mm Hg; heart rate, 85 beats/minute; respiratory rate, 22 breaths/minute). Staff members then connect him to an ECG monitor, which shows the following rhythm:

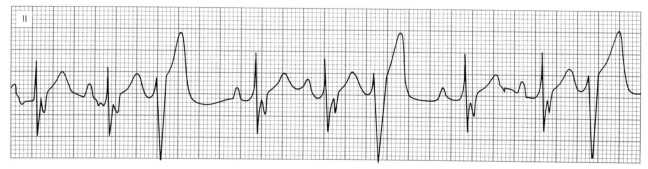

Interpret the rhythm, and list appropriate interventions for ED staff members to consider.

2. Mrs. M., age 76, weighs 110 lb (50 kg) and has a history of anterolateral myocardial infarction (MI). She was admitted to the coronary care unit (CCU) 2 hours ago for treatment of pulmonary edema. On admission, she received 0.5 mg of digoxin (Lanoxin) I.V. and 80 mg of furosemide (Lasix) I.V., and her ECG showed an atrial flutter with varying conduction and a ventricular rate of approximately 140 beats/minute. Oxygen is administered at 4 liters/minute by nasal cannula, and a patent I.V. line has been established. A nurse assigned to Mrs. M., after noting the rhythm change shown below, determines that Mrs. M. is pulseless and unresponsive:

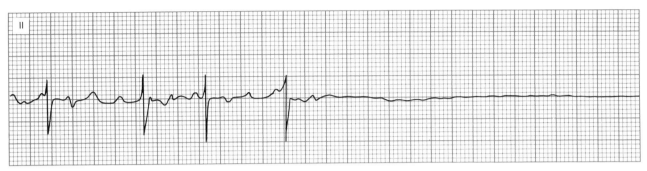

Interpret the rhythm, and list appropriate interventions to treat Mrs. M.'s condition.

3. After experiencing sudden palpitations and feeling dizzy at work, Mr. B., age 45, was transported to the ED by paramedics. En route, the paramedics started an I.V. infusion of dextrose 5% in water (D$_5$W) at a keep-vein-open rate and began administering oxygen by nasal cannula at 6 liters/minute. Now, Mr. B. appears pale, diaphoretic, and apprehensive as a nurse records his vital signs (blood pressure, 86/50 mm Hg; heart rate, 250 beats/minute; respiratory rate, 24 breaths/minute). Staff members then connect him to an ECG monitor, which shows the following rhythm:

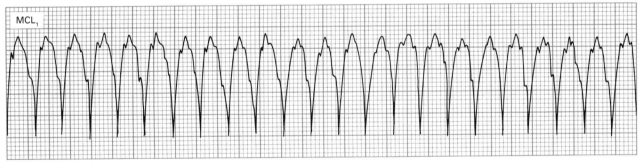

Interpret the rhythm, and list appropriate interventions to treat Mr. B.'s condition.

4. Mr. R., age 58, is being monitored in the telemetry unit for recurrence of premature ventricular complexes (PVCs), which had been controlled for the past 6 months with quinidine therapy. He is currently receiving maintenance doses of quinidine (200 mg four times daily). A nurse assigned to Mr. R. observes the following rhythm on the monitor:

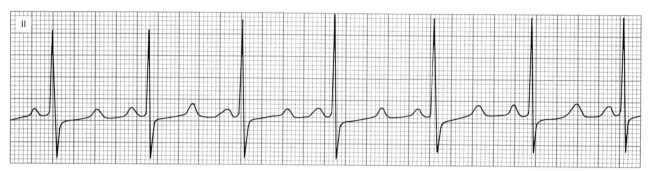

Interpret the rhythm (including estimates for the heart rate, PR interval, QRS complex duration, and QT interval), and list appropriate interventions for staff members to consider.

5. Mr. R. starts having more PVCs, including one that occurs on a T wave, producing the rhythm shown below. Mr. R. loses consciousness. The nurse cannot detect a pulse.

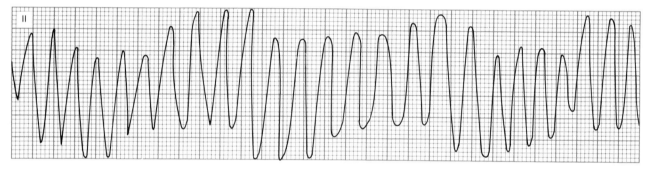

Interpret the rhythm, and list appropriate interventions to treat Mr. R.'s condition.

6. Paramedics arrive at the home of Mrs. F., age 64, in response to a 911 call from her daughter, who stated that Mrs. F. had passed out at the dinner table. In assessing Mrs. F., the paramedics can detect a slow pulse and note that she is lethargic, though responsive. Her daughter tells the paramedics that Mrs. F. has a history of syncopal episodes. They record her blood pressure (86/50 mm Hg), heart rate (25 beats/minute), and respiratory rate (14 breaths/minute) and connect her to an ECG monitor, which shows the following rhythm:

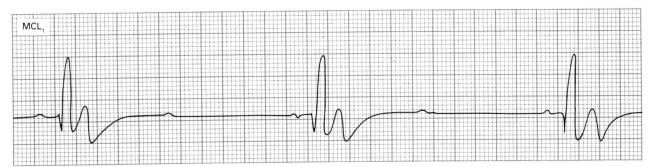

Interpret the rhythm, and discuss appropriate interventions for the paramedics to consider in treating Mrs. F.

7. Mr. C., age 65, was admitted to the CCU 12 hours ago for treatment of an inferior MI. He is connected to a cardiac monitor, oxygen is administered at 4 liters/minute via nasal cannula, and an I.V. heparin lock is in place. Mr. C., who weighs 176 lb (80 kg), complains of light-headedness to his assigned nurse, who records the following vital signs: blood pressure, 88/52 mm Hg; heart rate, 44 beats/minute; respiratory rate, 20 breaths/minute. On the ECG monitor, the following rhythm appears:

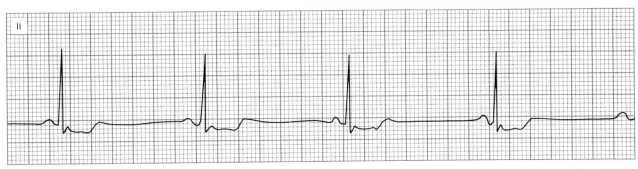

Interpret the rhythm, and state appropriate interventions for CCU staff members to initiate.

8. Friends of Mr. K., age 25, bring him to the ED after he falls onto the roadway from the back of a slow-moving pickup truck. On arrival, he is pulseless and unresponsive. He has abrasions on his forearms and chest but no obvious deformities or fractures. The ECG monitor shows the following rhythm:

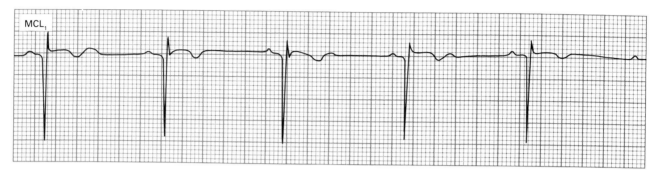

Interpret the rhythm, and discuss appropriate interventions for the ED staff to initiate.

9. Mr. T., age 60 and weighing 198 lb (90 kg), is admitted to the hospital's telemetry unit for treatment of syncopal episodes associated with "skipped beats." An I.V. heparin lock is in place. Mr. T. is walking without difficulty in the hallway when a nurse, viewing the cardiac monitor at the nurse's station, observes the rhythm shown here:

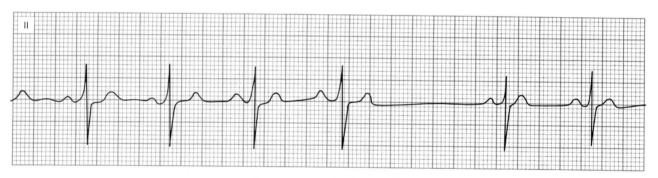

Interpret the rhythm, and list appropriate interventions for staff members to initiate.

10. Mr. Y., age 58 and weighing 220 lb (100 kg), is being treated in the CCU for an anteroseptal MI. His blood pressure is 84/52 mm Hg; heart rate, 36 beats/minute; respiratory rate, 18 breaths/minute. An I.V. infusion of D_5W is flowing at a keep-vein-open rate, and oxygen is being administered at 6 liters/minute. Additionally, Mr. Y. has received a total of 2 mg of atropine I.V. in response to the rhythm shown below, which began suddenly about 20 minutes ago.

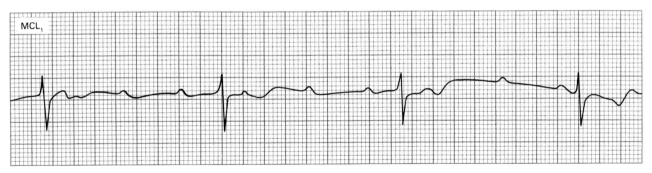

Interpret the rhythm, and list appropriate interventions to treat Mr. Y.'s condition.

11. Mr. L., age 42, is being treated in the CCU for severe substernal chest pain radiating to his left shoulder and neck. An I.V. infusion of D_5W is flowing at a keep-vein-open rate, and oxygen is being administered via nasal cannula at 5 liters/minute. Mr. L., who weighs 165 lb (75 kg), has had a few isolated PVCs. Just moments ago, after a nurse recorded his blood pressure (140/88 mm Hg), heart rate (96 beats/minute), and respiratory rate (20 breaths/minute), he told her that his heart felt as if it were "flipping over," and the following rhythm appeared on the monitor:

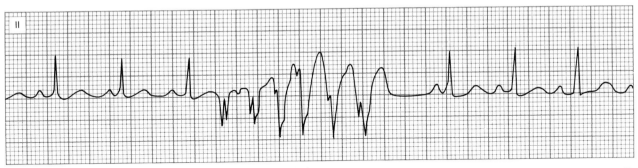

Interpret the rhythm, and describe interventions that the CCU staff should initiate.

12. Mrs. A., age 38, comes to the ED after feeling chest pressure that has persisted for 6 hours. She appears anxious and apprehensive when describing her symptoms to the admitting nurse, stating that, on a scale of 1 to 10, her pain is currently an 8. Noting that Mrs. A. is pale and diaphoretic, the nurse records her weight (88 lb [40 kg]) and vital signs (blood pressure, 90/62 mm Hg; heart rate, 135 beats/minute; respiratory rate, 24 breaths/minute). ED staff members then connect her to a cardiac monitor, which shows the following rhythm:

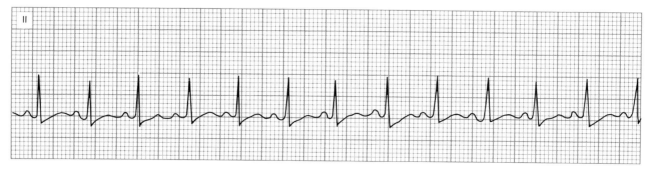

Interpret the rhythm, and list appropriate interventions for the staff to consider in treating Mrs. A.'s condition.

13. Mr. J., age 58, is in the cardiology clinic for a routine evaluation of his DDD pacemaker. He is asymptomatic. His blood pressure is 128/86 mm Hg; heart rate, 72 beats/minute; respiratory rate, 16 breaths/minute. The cardiac monitor shows the following rhythm:

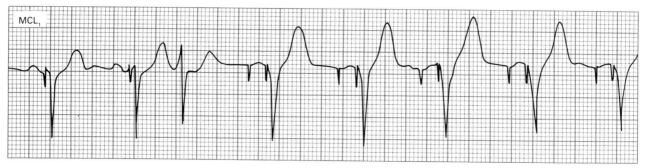

Interpret the rhythm, and discuss appropriate interventions.

14. Mrs. D., age 78, is being treated in the CCU for an anterolateral MI. She is receiving oxygen by nasal cannula at 4 liters/minute and 0.25 mg of digoxin as a daily maintenance dose. Her blood pressure is 130/86 mm Hg; heart rate, 56 beats/minute; and respiratory rate, 20 breaths/minute. The ECG monitor shows the following rhythm:

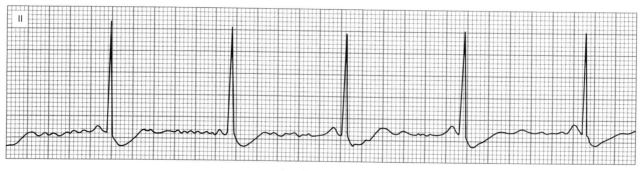

Interpret the rhythm, and identify appropriate interventions.

15. Jessica S., 3 weeks old, is brought to the ED by her parents, who are concerned because Jessica has been unable to breast-feed properly and seems lethargic. A nurse records Jessica's weight (7 lb [3 kg]), blood pressure (60 mm Hg), heart rate (270 beats/minute), and respiratory rate (50 breaths/minute, with bilateral breath sounds). Staff members then connect Jessica to a cardiac monitor, which shows the following rhythm:

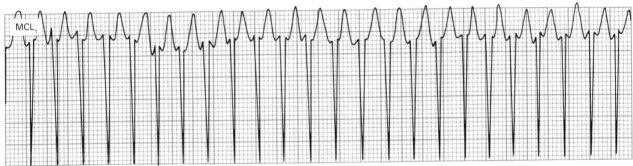

Interpret the rhythm, and discuss appropriate interventions to treat Jessica's condition.

16. Mr. N., age 59 and weighing 220 lb (100 kg), is a patient in the hospital's transitional care unit. Having a history of atrial fibrillation, he has been taking 0.25 mg of digoxin daily for the last 4 years. While a nurse records his blood pressure (124/78 mm Hg), heart rate (35 beats/minute), and respiratory rate (18 breaths/minute), Mr. N. says that he has not felt well for the last week and his appetite has diminished. The ECG monitor shows the following rhythm:

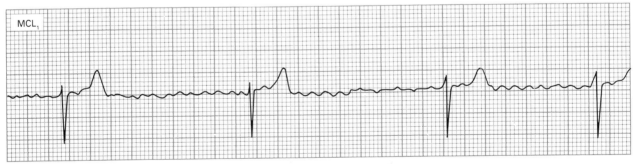

Interpret the rhythm, and list appropriate interventions to treat Mr. N.'s condition.

17. Mrs. W., age 80, is admitted to the telemetry unit with congestive heart failure. A nurse records her blood pressure (90/58 mm Hg), heart rate (120 beats/minute), and respiratory rate (32 breaths/

minute), noting that Mrs. W. has bilateral rales at the lung bases and appears to be breathing with great difficulty. On the ECG monitor, the following rhythm appears:

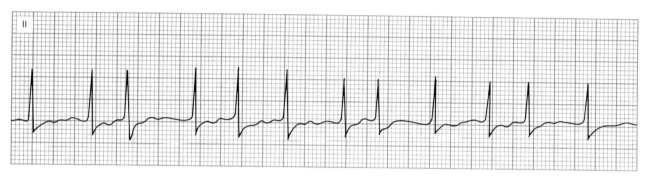

Interpret the rhythm, and discuss appropriate interventions for staff members to initiate.

18. Mr. P., age 78 and weighing about 165 lb (75 kg), is pulseless and unresponsive when paramedics bring him to the ED. With cardiopulmonary resuscitation (CPR) in progress, the paramedics report that three defibrillations have failed to change Mr. P.'s rhythm. They have already begun an I.V. infusion of D_5W. Mr. P.'s rhythm is shown here:

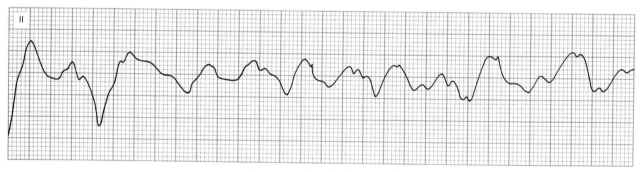

Interpret the rhythm, and list appropriate interventions to treat Mr. P.'s condition.

19. Mr. H., age 47, is recuperating in the CCU after suffering an anterior-wall MI. About 10 minutes ago, a nurse recorded his blood pressure (138/86 mm Hg), heart rate (66 beats/minute), and respiratory rate (16 breaths/minute). Mr. H. is currently free from pain. The ECG shows the following rhythm:

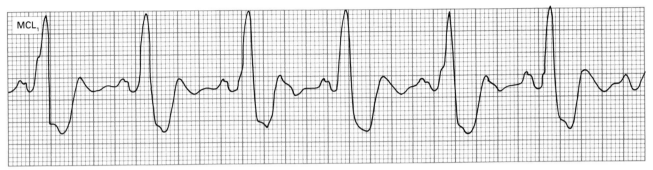

Interpret the rhythm, and identify appropriate interventions to consider.

Answers to self-test

1. *Rhythm interpretation*
   Sinus rhythm with ventricular trigeminy (every third complex is a premature ventricular complex [PVC])

   Interventions
   • Administer oxygen at 4 to 6 liters/minute via nasal cannula or face mask.
   • Start an I.V. infusion of dextrose 5% in water (D_5W).
   • Administer 70 mg of lidocaine (Xylocaine) by I.V. bolus. Repeat half this dose (35 mg) every 2 to 5 minutes, up to a total dosage of 210 mg (3 mg/kg).
   • Administer 2 to 5 mg of morphine sulfate I.V. or 0.3 to 0.4 mg of nitroglycerin (Nitrostat) sublingually.

2. *Rhythm interpretation*
   Atrial flutter with varying conduction (3:1 and 4:1) to asystole

   Interventions
   • Call a code.
   • Begin and maintain cardiopulmonary resuscitation (CPR).
   • Administer 1 mg of epinephrine (Adrenalin) I.V.
   • Initiate endotracheal intubation.
   • If the rhythm does not change, administer 1 mg of atropine I.V.
   • If the rhythm does not change, consider an external or transvenous pacemaker.

3. *Rhythm interpretation*
   Unstable supraventricular tachycardia (probably paroxysmal, given the patient's symptoms on admission)

   Interventions
   • Prepare for cardioversion.
   • Administer 5 mg of diazepam (Valium) or 2 to 2.5 mg of midazolam (Versed) I.V.

- Institute cardioversion at 100 joules.
- If the rhythm does not change, repeat at 200 joules.
- If the rhythm does not change, repeat at 360 joules.
- Correct underlying abnormalities, such as hypoxemia.
- Initiate pharmacologic therapy with verapamil (Calan), propranolol (Inderal), or esmolol (Brevibloc).

4. *Rhythm interpretation*
Sinus rhythm with a heart rate of 66 beats/minute, a PR interval of 0.18 second, a QRS complex duration of 0.10 second, and a QT interval of 0.44 second

Interventions
- Observe for further lengthening of the QT interval (0.44 second is abnormally long for this heart rate).
- Consider the possibility of quinidine (Quinidex) toxicity. Order appropriate laboratory studies and discontinue quinidine, if indicated.

5. *Rhythm interpretation*
Torsades de pointes, a form of ventricular tachycardia (in this case, pulseless VT)

Interventions
- Administer a precordial thump.
- Call a code.
- Begin CPR.
- Defibrillate at 200 joules.
- If the rhythm does not change and the patient remains pulseless, repeat at 200 to 300 joules.
- If the rhythm does not change and the patient remains pulseless, repeat at 360 joules.
- If the rhythm does not change, resume CPR.
- Establish an I.V. line (if not already done).
- Administer 1 mg of epinephrine I.V.
- Initiate endotracheal intubation.
- Defibrillate at 360 joules.

6. *Rhythm interpretation*
Second-degree atrioventricular (AV) block Type II and right bundle branch block (RBBB)

Interventions
- Administer oxygen via nasal cannula at 6 liters/minute.
- Establish an I.V. line.
- Infuse D_5W, and consider administering a fluid bolus.
- Administer 1 mg of atropine I.V.
- If the rhythm does not change, administer 0.5 mg of atropine I.V.

every 5 minutes, up to a total dosage of 2 mg.
• Transport the patient to the emergency department (where the physician will probably consider inserting a pacemaker).

7. *Rhythm interpretation*
Sinus bradycardia

Interventions
• Increase the oxygen level to 6 liters/minute.
• Start an I.V. infusion of D_5W at a keep-vein-open rate.
• Administer 0.5 mg of atropine I.V. Repeat every 5 minutes, up to a total dosage of 2 mg.
• Consider administering a fluid challenge.
• Initiate pacemaker therapy if the above interventions fail and the patient remains symptomatic.

8. *Rhythm interpretation*
Sinus bradycardia with electromechanical dissociation (EMD), possibly secondary

Interventions
• Begin CPR. (When opening the patient's airway, take precautions to avoid neck injury.)
• Establish an I.V. line.
• Administer 1 mg of epinephrine I.V.
• Initiate endotracheal intubation.
• Administer a fluid challenge.
• Check the patient for other causes of EMD, such as pneumothorax (deviated trachea, lack of breath sounds on one side), cardiac tamponade (distended neck veins), acidosis, and hypoxemia (hyperventilate with 100% oxygen).

9. *Rhythm interpretation*
Sinus rhythm with one sinus pause caused by a sinoatrial block

Interventions
• Assess the patient. If he has no symptoms and vital signs are stable, no treatment is indicated.
• If he becomes symptomatic, administer 0.5 mg of atropine I.V. Repeat every 5 minutes, up to a total dosage of 2 mg.
• If symptoms persist, initiate pacemaker therapy.

10. *Rhythm interpretation*
Third-degree AV block (complete heart block)

Interventions
• Use an external pacemaker, if available.
• Administer isoproterenol (Isuprel), 2 to 10 mcg/minute, as a temporary measure.

•Insert a transvenous pacemaker.

11. *Rhythm interpretation*
Sinus rhythm with a nonsustained episode of VT (possibly torsades de pointes)

Interventions
•Administer 75 mg of lidocaine I.V. (If ectopy recurs, repeat lidocaine 37 mg I.V. every 2 to 5 minutes.)
•When ectopy resolves, start an I.V. drip of lidocaine at 2 to 4 mg/minute.
•Check the patient's serum potassium level (hypokalemia may cause this arrhythmia).

12. *Rhythm interpretation*
Sinus tachycardia

Interventions
•Administer oxygen at 4 to 6 liters/minute by nasal cannula.
•Start an I.V. infusion of D_5W at a keep-vein-open rate.
•Administer 2 to 5 mg of morphine sulfate I.V. or 3 to 4 mg of nitroglycerin sublingually.
•Reassess the patient's vital signs.
•Obtain a 12-lead ECG.

13. *Rhythm interpretation*
Correctly functioning DDD pacemaker (The first three beats are atrial-triggered, ventricular-paced; the fourth is a PVC; the remainder are atrial- and ventricular-paced. The AV interval is 0.16 second.)

Interventions
•Assess for palpable pulses to ensure that all paced beats are perfusing.

14. *Rhythm interpretation*
Sinus bradycardia with artifact from muscle movement or loose electrodes

Interventions
•Check for loose electrodes, which can cause the artifact.
•Treat bradycardia only if the patient becomes symptomatic (hypotension, altered level of consciousness, PVCs).

15. *Rhythm interpretation*
Supraventricular tachycardia

Interventions
•Administer low-flow oxygen by cannula or hood.
•Start an I.V. line.

•Institute cardioversion at 3 joules. (If ineffective, repeat at 6 joules.)
•If cardioversion is ineffective, consider administering digoxin (Lanoxin). (An infant's reaction to digoxin is highly individualized. A suggested initial dose is 30 to 35 mcg/kg.)

16. *Rhythm interpretation*
Atrial fibrillation with a slow ventricular response

Interventions
•Administer oxygen at 4 to 6 liters/minute by nasal cannula.
•Check the patient's serum potassium and digoxin levels. His symptoms indicate possible digoxin toxicity.
•Refer to the bradycardia algorithm (page 155) if the patient develops more symptoms.

17. *Rhythm interpretation*
Atrial fibrillation with a fast ventricular response

Interventions
•Administer oxygen at 4 to 6 liters/minute by nasal cannula.
•Start an I.V. infusion of D_5W.
•Administer 0.25 mg of digoxin I.V. or institute cardioversion.
•Administer 20 to 80 mg of furosemide (Lasix).

18. *Rhythm interpretation*
Ventricular fibrillation

Interventions
•Reassess the patient and continue CPR.
•Administer 1 mg of epinephrine, 1:10,000 I.V. (Additional doses of 1 to 5 mg may be administered every 5 minutes.)
•Initiate endotracheal intubation.
•Defibrillate with 360 joules.
•Reassess the patient.
•Administer 75 mg of lidocaine I.V.
•Defibrillate with 360 joules.
•Consider administering sodium bicarbonate or bretylium (Bretylol).

19. *Rhythm interpretation*
Sinus rhythm with RBBB

Interventions
•Continue to monitor the patient.
•Check a 12-lead ECG for signs of anterior or posterior fascicular block, such as an axis deviation and typical QRS configurations in leads III and aV_L.

Selected References

Albarran-Sotelo, R., et al. *Textbook of Advanced Cardiac Life Support,* 2nd ed. Dallas: American Heart Association, 1987.

Andreoli, R., et al. *Cecil Essentials of Medicine,* 2nd ed. Philadelphia: W.B. Saunders Co., 1989.

Bartz, C. "Pharmacologic Augmentation of Cardiac Output Following Cardiac Arrest," *Critical Care Nursing Quarterly* 10(4):43-49, March 1988.

Callaham, M. "Advances in the Management of Cardiac Arrest," *Western Journal of Medicine* 145(5):670-75, November 1986.

Cardiovascular Care Handbook. Springhouse, Pa.: Springhouse Corp., 1986.

Chameides, L., ed. *Textbook of Pediatric Advanced Life Support.* Dallas: American Heart Association and American Academy of Pediatrics, 1988.

EKG Cards. Springhouse, Pa.: Springhouse Corp., 1987.

Garrett, A.E., and Adams, V. *Pocket Handbook of Common Cardiac Arrhythmias: Recognition and Treatment.* Philadelphia: J.B. Lippincott Co., 1986.

Gikonyo, B.M., et al. "Cardiovascular Collapse in Infants: Association with Paroxysmal Atrial Tachycardia," *Pediatrics* 76(6):922-26, December 1985.

Gonzalez, E.R., et al. "Dose-Dependent Vasopressor Response to Epinephrine during CPR in Human Beings," *Annals of Emergency Medicine* 18(9):920-26, September 1989.

Goodwin, B.A. "Pediatric Resuscitation," *Critical Care Nursing Quarterly* 10(4):69-79, March 1988.

Guyton, A.C. *Textbook of Medical Physiology,* 7th ed. Philadelphia: W.B. Saunders Co., 1986.

Holloway, N. *Nursing the Critically Ill Adult,* 3rd ed. Menlo Park, Calif.: Addison-Wesley Publishing Co., 1988.

Jaffe, A.S. "Cardiovascular Pharmacology, Part I," *Circulation* 74(6, Pt. 2) IV 70-74, December 1986.

Jost, P. "The Role of Antidysrhythmics in Cardiac Arrest," *Critical Care Nursing Quarterly* 10(4):63-67, March 1988.

Kim, H.S., and Chung, E.K. "Torsades de Pointes: Polymorphous Ventricular Tachycardia," *Heart and Lung* 12(3):269-73, May 1983.

Middaugh, R.E., et al. "Current Considerations in Respiratory and Acid-Base Management during Cardiopulmonary Resuscitation," *Critical Care Nursing Quarterly* 10(4):25-33, March 1988.

Montgomery, W.H. "Standards and Guidelines for Cardiopulmonary Resuscitation and Emergency Cardiac Care," *Circulation* 74(6, Pt. 2) IV 1-3, December 1986.

Otto, C.W. "Cardiovascular Pharmacology, Part II: The Use of Catecholamines, Pressor Agents, Digitalis, and Corticosteroids in CPR and Emergency Cardiac Care," *Circulation* 74(6, Pt. 2) IV 80-85, December 1986.

Paraskos, J.A. "Cardiovascular Pharmacology, Part III: Atropine, Calcium, Calcium Blockers, and Beta-Blockers," *Circulation* 74(6, Pt. 2) IV 86-89, December 1986.

Scherer, P. "ACLS Guidelines: What Nurses Are Saying about the Drug Changes," *American Journal of Nursing* 86(12):1352-58, December 1986.

"Standards and Guidelines for Cardiopulmonary Resuscitation (CPR) and Emergency Cardiac Care (ECC)," *JAMA* 255(21):2905-84, June 6, 1986.

Swearingen, P., et al., eds. *Manual of Critical Care: Applying Nursing Diagnoses to Adult Critical Illnesses,* 2nd ed. St. Louis: C.V. Mosby Co., 1991.

Weaver, W.D. "Calcium-Channel Blockers and Advanced Cardiac Life Support," *Circulation* 74(6, Pt. 2) IV 94-97, December 1986.

Index

i refers to an illustration; t refers to a table.